Advancing Technology, Caring, and Nursing

EDITED BY

Rozzano C. Locsin

AUBURN HOUSE
Westport, Connecticut • London

Library of Congress Cataloging-in-Publication Data

Advancing technology, caring, and nursing / edited by Rozzano C. Locsin.
   p. cm.
   Includes bibliographical references and index.
   ISBN 0–86569–300–5 (alk. paper)—ISBN 0–86569–302–1 (pbk. : alk. paper)
   1. Nursing. 2. Empathy. 3. Technology. I. Locsin, Rozzano C., 1954–
   [DNLM: 1. Nursing Care. 2. Empathy. 3. Technology. WY 100 A2446 2001]
  RT42.A345 2001
  610.73—dc21   00–045393

British Library Cataloguing in Publication Data is available.

Library of Congress Catalog Card Number: 00–045393
ISBN: 0–86569–300–5 (hc)
     0–86569–302–1 (pb)

First published in 2001

Auburn House, 88 Post Road West, Westport, CT 06881
An imprint of Greenwood Publishing Group, Inc.
www.greenwood.com

Printed in the United States of America

The paper used in this book complies with the
Permanent Paper Standard issued by the National
Information Standards Organization (Z39.48–1984).

10 9 8 7 6 5 4 3 2 1

My father wanted me to be a nurse. I am a nurse now. He has passed on. This book is for him—in memoriam. He would have been very proud. It is an accomplishment of his son. I miss him. He directed my life—now he is my star.

Contents

Foreword

Jean Watson

There are few books which are published just in time to help solve some of the pressing dilemmas of an era. *Advancing Technology, Caring, and Nursing* is such a book. The realities, ambiguities, and controls of science, technology, and human experiences are turned upside down and inside out as the postmodern condition of this new millennium races toward us. Efforts to sustain human caring during such a chaotic era in history remind us that technology and machines have entered more quickly into our personal and professional lives than we have been able to move toward them, or assimilate them into the human experience. Thus, we see why a book that helps us to conceptualize, critique, and re-create our proper relationship between the three is needed and comes just in time. Nursing is in the precarious position of possibly not making it through this new century unless it shifts its discourse and clarifies its professional ethic and informed moral actions to sustain caring in nursing, and simultaneously acknowledges the emergence of a new relationship to the human-technology interface as a central tenet of professional nursing.

In addition to the new, emerging relationships between humans and technology, we also see the smaller universe unfolding, a universe that, ironically, brings humans closer to humans. Through non-contact touch of machines and breakthroughs in consciousness, and new theories of how humans evolve and co-evolve in continuous relationship to this new human-technology phenomenon, we are led to paradoxical possibilities of deepening depersonalization, as well as deepening human connections. This work is a critical text for nursing scholars in that it reflects upon the dilemmas and possibilities for sustaining caring and humanity in the midst of technological evolution. This effort is one of the seminal calls for nursing and health professionals to address during this era of human history. This text helps to integrate the paradox and complexities of cultural changes. Along with a humanitarian ethic, relating human and technological connections with a global concern, it offers a healthy dialectic for the technological-caring dilemma.

It is not that technology is bad in and of itself, as we know and live with its benefits; it is, however, necessary to critique and discern the dramatic and subtle impact and evolution, as well as the potential erosion of human caring, that can occur without reflection and professional pause. As technology moves to the foreground, human caring and the human experience itself often move to the background, removing humans from the center of their own existence and detouring the practitioner from the human aspects of caring toward care for (and attention diverted toward) machines.

Further, as more and more technology dominates the consciousness of both patient and practitioner, both nurse and patient are potentially reduced to the moral status of object. Since one person's level of humanity is reflected upon another, when one is reduced to object status morally, and often even physically or psychologically, so is the other. Another consequence of this slippery slope of unleashed technology without critique and reflection is that, when the human is reduced from fully human (and humane) status, consciously or unconsciously, we set up circumstances whereby one can justify manipulating and controlling another, or doing something to another as object that one would not do were that person to be adamantly sustained as fully human.

Just as the dangers are there, demanding consideration, so are dramatic possibilities of a new era of human-to-human communication and connection that emerge through this new human-technology interface. For example, some of the tenets of contemporary caring science models suggest such notions that caring (consciousness) transcends time, space, and physicality. Such thinking opens new views of caring technology, allowing for virtual caring to be communicated across time and space (Watson, 1999). With this new thinking of a caring science–technology interface, technology can be reframed as connecting humans rather than separating them. (Witness the revolution in Internet relationships and the development of virtual communities of persons who share common life events.) The limits of the new connections between caring and technology are unknown and unlimited. Thus, these works offer an occasion to pause, to reflect, and to rethink the very notions of technology, caring, nursing, and the human condition.

These and other pressing issues are the focus of this important text, which offers informed and discerning pause and reflection, as well as exploration of these knotty dynamics and dialectics of the evolving human, technological, caring universe of a new world. If we take this next turn in technology, caring, and nursing seriously enough, we just may end up considering human caring as the foundation for the metaphysics of virtual reality (Heim, 1993) as well as the discipline of nursing, thus awakening us to the fact that we are in the middle of redefining technology, caring, and nursing itself. This turn and this text point the way toward this future that awaits, unfolding in time and space, real and virtual.

REFERENCES

Heim, M. (1993). *The metaphysics of virtual reality*. Oxford: Oxford University Press.

Watson, J. (1999). *Postmodern nursing and beyond*. New York: Churchill-Livingstone/Harcourt Brace.

Preface

The nurse who is technologically proficient is often perceived as a nurse who is not caring. Because technological competency is often understood as the defining description of contemporary nursing practice, it serves as the primary influence in understanding nursing as a valuable health care practice. Regardless of practice settings, nurses lament the lack of time to care—often attributed to the critical expectation of achieving technological competency, as if caring is a separate entity that needs to be accomplished in addition to being technologically competent. With this understanding, the assertion is made that being technologically competent is being caring.

The purpose of this book is to provide learned expositions of issues regarding the harmonious coexistence of technology and caring—concepts integral to the valuable practice of nursing as essential to health and well-being. A multi-contributed book was believed to be the best way to lay bare understandings and encourage dialogue about fundamental concepts of the two seemingly dichotomous concepts of technology and caring in nursing. The variety of issues and subjects spanning a single concern—that of explicating the harmonious coexistence of technology and caring in nursing—provided the impetus to contribute to this book.

Topics that provoke and motivate intellectual discourse establish the differing sections of the book, from foundational issues of caring in contemporary nursing, including influences of technology like machines, language, application, and practice issues, to "telehealth" and ethico-moral consequences of technology and caring in nursing. In addressing these topics, contributors were asked to submit manuscripts about topics they have always considered crucial to articulating the relationships among technology, caring, and nursing.

While concerns for technological advances create stirring issues about caring and nursing, it is particularly important to consider the understanding that while technologies change, competency expressed as caring in nursing does not.

The intended audience for the book is broad. It includes basic and advanced students of nursing, practicing professional nurses, academicians, and other health care personnel who can benefit from thought-provoking discussions about the seemingly dichotomous concepts of technology and caring in nursing. A discourse such as this facilitates the meaningful understanding of the influence of technology on health care, and, in particular, on nursing practice.

This book can be used as a text in schools and colleges of nursing for courses such as basic nursing courses introducing professional nursing, health care administration courses, critical care nursing courses, and courses focusing on transformations of contemporary nursing practices. Of particular value is the salience of the book for the study and practice of advanced nursing in technological competency, as caring in nursing assumes a primary role.

In the Introduction, the stage is set for a scholarly and practical discourse initiated by a description of the valuing of the concepts of technology, caring, and nursing. The first of three parts provides chapters that focus on the foundational concepts of caring in nursing and technology in nursing. Issues relevant to application of these concepts, including ethico-moral considerations of practice, comprise the second and third parts.

The editor hopes that the valuable insights derived from the visions portrayed in this book will stimulate thought and move discourse toward recognizing, understanding, and realizing the value of technological competency as the contemporary expression of nursing practice grounded in caring.

Acknowledgments

This is to acknowledge the authors who have contributed to this book, experts in nursing who share my passion for continuing dialogue on the influences of technology and caring coexisting in nursing. While I have known most of the contributors personally, some I have only known through cyber connections—the technology of the Internet. Nevertheless, even with such a potentially impersonal medium, I feel we know each other well through our mutual fondness for nursing and its scholarship.

The publication of this book was inspired by the challenges posited by technological advances on nursing as a discipline of knowledge, and a practice profession. In editing a multi-contributed book, finding a publisher you can work with, and the unwavering commitment and perseverance of the contributors are essential.

This acknowledgment also goes to the one who always walks with me, without whom my endeavors would be fruitless and insignificant—always there with me in unique ways.

My appreciation for technological competency as an expression of caring in nursing continues to be nurtured through the mentorship of Dr. Savina Schoenhofer, who continues to challenge me, and Marguerite Purnell, through her love of nursing and scholarly endeavors.

To all current and future nurses, I challenge you to continue to discover ways of expressing nursing as a responsive, creative, and innovative health care practice and as a discipline of knowledge.

Introduction

Rozzano C. Locsin

The complexities of technology intimately touch aspects of nursing in every setting. These complexities continue to challenge the appreciation of nursing as a professional practice that is both integral and valuable to health care. The prominence of caring as the central focus of nursing is acknowledged through the generation of theories and frameworks that guide its practice. The understanding of caring as not unique to nursing, but *in* nursing, expresses the thematic discourse that continues to excite scholars and practitioners of nursing. Nevertheless, the question relative to praxis continues to be asked: "How is caring practiced uniquely in nursing?" Ways of expressing modes of caring in nursing are being deliberately challenged.

Technological competency defines contemporary nursing practice. Varying descriptions and definitions of technology have generated this definition. The popular understanding of technology as any factor which influences efficiency has become the primary criterion for discerning the use and value of technology. Often, technological proficiency describes excellent nurses. How do these nurses competently use technology such that competence becomes the defining characteristic of their excellence in practice? It is clear that being technologically proficient alone can make the performance of tasks an excellent practice of nursing. However, the debate over nursing practice characterized as completion of tasks dominates nursing practice forums. Many non-nurses—technicians—perform tasks efficiently and proficiently. However, the advent of high-tech machines and the ascription of technological competency as the major criterion for defining who and what is a nurse make nurses appear more as technologists (and as their non-nurse counterparts) than as knowledgeable, professional practitioners of nursing. A vital ingredient in the recognition of nursing as a knowledgeable practice is the use of technologies in the process of knowing persons in their wholeness. Such an appreciation epitomizes the proficient use of technology for the ultimate purpose of acknowledging persons in their wholeness. So, while technology may bring the nurse closer to the patient through performing technological tasks, paradoxically, technology also provides the chance for the nurse to disregard the person as a human being. A mechanistic view of human beings allows for the appreciation of persons as made up of distinct parts. This view of persons is the antithesis of the human science view, in which humans are distinguished as whole and complete, and therefore do not need to be fixed or to be made whole again.

TECHNOLOGICAL EXPRESSIONS

"It is appallingly clear that our technology has surpassed our humanity." Attributed to Albert Einstein in the movie *Powder* (1995), this commentary on a perceived inverse relationship between technology and humanity may seem justified. Referring to this same statement, Jeremy Reese, the character of the movie, was fittingly attributed this meaningful remark, "I look at you and I think that someday, our humanity may actually surpass our technology" (*Powder*, 1995). While dependency on technology may define our way of living as ordinary existence, a hopeful intention is to recognize that, eventually, being human may actually transcend dependency on technology. The value in addressing being human as a hoped-for persona, rather than technology, is inestimable.

This book is about technology, caring, and nursing. The word "technology" originated from two Greek concepts: *logos*, relating to the rational order of things, and *techne*, the know-how of making things. While know-how can refer to the process or procedure of making things, techne as knowing may be better understood when described by the phrase "know-that." While the word "how" may refer to a process, when combined with "know," it simply unravels to mean a well-constructed description of crucial information. The popular understanding of "know-how" is its reference to the instance of purposive and intentional application.

Several definitions of technology exist, but one fits nursing well. To Heidegger (1977), technology is a means to an end; an instrument as well as a human activity. Consider the electrocardiogram, a technological instrument that exhibits data showing the cardiac activity of a living human being. Interpreting the accumulated data from this instrument is a human activity. The data derived provide information which forms the bases for medical and nursing care technologies essential to maintaining patients' health (Locsin, 1995). The answer to the question, "Why is nursing practice popularly understood as simply proficiency with technologies?" is of critical importance. In this book, the stream of intention is to recognize and understand that technological competency *is* an expression of caring in nursing.

Various technologies exist that exemplify a particulate relationship with humanity, and a certain valuing of the mechanistic view. Future technologies that may influence health care may take the shape of a chemically created computer in the form of a molecule. This molecular computer may insert itself as "tiny probes in the body, . . . monitor body functions—perhaps a very sophisticated pacemaker." Currently, a molecular computer exists that is called the Chemically-Assembled Electronic Nanocomputers or CAENs (*Palm Beach Post*, July 17, 1999). This technology is an example of the relatedness and dependency that currently exist between technology and being human.

The influence of technological developments gave rise to increased discourse in nursing literature focused on the effects of technology on human beings. Dean (1998) portrayed the combination of technical proficiency, scientific knowledge, and nursing artistry, which can still preserve the humanity and dignity of patients and their relatives in a critical care environment. Even with the proliferation of medical technologies in health care and the increasing dependence upon technology for regulation and ordering of tasks, nursing continues to inspire the evolution of a practice perspective: that of valuing persons in their wholeness.

Currently, varying descriptions of nursing (a consequence of "shifting paradigms" and philosophies of science) create differing views of caring, such as caring being the essence of nursing (Leininger, 1988), the human mode of being (Roach, 1984), and the moral ideal of nursing (Watson, 1985). These caring perspectives influence the perceptions of who is a caring person; for example, a human being who expresses caring ingredients (Mayeroff, 1971), and one who exhibits attributes of caring (Roach, 1984). Boykin and Schoenhofer (1993) declared the centrality of caring in nursing. This declaration affirms that "all nursing takes place in nursing situations, the shared lived experience in which the caring between nurse and the one nursed, enhances personhood" (p. 23). Consequently, the ultimate purpose of technological competency in nursing is the conscious acknowledgment of persons as human beings who are complete in the moment, and do not need any fixing.

Advancing Technology, Caring, and Nursing is a book that provides scholars of nursing, nursing practitioners, students of basic and advanced nursing, and other health care professionals the opportunity to enhance their appreciation and participation in contemporary discourse about the dominant position technology has attained in the mainstream world of health care. This book aims to clarify the valuing of two seemingly dichotomous concepts: those of technology and of caring in nursing. The design is intended to bring forward examination of the continuing domination of health care technologies in contemporary nursing practice. Using caring as the lens through which nursing practice can be advanced continues to challenge contemporary practice.

While technology in health care is primarily described as machines and equipment, other views exist, such as diverse technologies of representation and control, language, and personification from European and American perspectives. These realities make the influence of technology on nursing and its practice necessarily integral for a sustainable and globalized health care. Further, together with the prevailing and sensitive issues of telehealth, advances in genetics and cloning, and nanotechnologies, the dependency of health care on technologies takes on a central position.

Technocratic issues, such as high-tech home care and the revolution of prescribing patient care based on institution patient-day stays, support and incite the inclusion of practices and concerns that are relevant to non-critical care settings. Ultimately, this book should challenge the readers to rethink contemporary health care, globalization in health care, and health care dependency on technology.

KNOWING PERSONS IN THEIR WHOLENESS

By embracing technology, caring, and nursing as themes of the book, emphases were placed on the dominance of technology in health care, the centrality of caring in nursing, and the understanding of nursing as a discipline of knowledge and a professional practice. From these themes evolved the concept of technological competency as an expression of caring in nursing—the illustration of nursing practice predicated upon the understanding of persons in their wholeness. The ultimate purpose of technological competency in nursing is the conscious acknowledgment of persons in their wholeness, and it directs the practice of using technologies of nursing to "know" persons as human beings, rather than as objects. Knowing persons' wholeness discourages the objectification of human beings that often (perhaps unintentionally) plagues the practice of high-tech nurses. It is the intention of the nurse that facilitates the realization of what is nursing. From the lens of "intention to nurse," nursing practitioners recognize patients as human beings who are complete and therefore do not need any fixing (Boykin & Schoenhofer, 1993; Purnell & Locsin, 2000). To high-tech, critical care nurses whose expertise is the one, true, meaningful way they can know persons in their wholeness, technological competency is an expression of caring in nursing.

The concern is not how the nurse knows the patient, but rather, why the nurse wants to know and why the nurse wants to use specific technologies. For what reason is a particular process of nursing of interest to the nurse whose practice centers on knowing persons in their wholeness? Knowing persons in their wholeness is a conceptualization of a nursing process in which a mutual, simultaneous, authentic, and deliberate practice of nursing is appreciated: The concept of persons in their wholeness is the foundation from which technological competency as expression of caring in nursing lives.

While RN's may be legally required to supervise intravenous medicine administration, a cheaper provider should do as many of the more menial tasks as possible. A cheaper someone else can give the pills. A cheaper someone else can feed the patient. A cheaper someone else can give the bath. The patient's vital signs may be on a clipboard somewhere, recorded by some cheaper observer, and often correctly noted. Yet, nobody knows the patient. Respirations, 32, Temperature 102, Pulse 36. All accurate data. But why these particular values? Do they signify anything? How about the patient? The patient? (Shragg, 1995, p. 5)

Mitchell (1995) has consistently argued that through nursing diagnosis, the patient is made known from a Cartesian dualistic perspective of mind and body, rather than as one who is whole and complete in the moment. The popular nursing process of assessing body systems and organs, establishing a nursing diagnosis, and the implementation of actions predicted from the patient's status of physiological functioning is living nursing from the perspective of the biomedical, mechanistic model. Practicing nursing from this viewpoint sustains and reinforces the view of persons as a composite of various parts. Contrary to this recognition is the process of knowing persons in their wholeness. The recognition of this process is described as the intentional and reciprocal "coming to know persons" as complete in the moment. Counter to the reductionist perspective, knowing persons in their wholeness allows for the celebration of the uniqueness, irreducibility, and unpredictability of human beings (Locsin, 1997). In essence, the nurse and the nursed participate in mutual recognition of their wholeness as a foundation for growth within the intimacy of the nursing relationship.

Knowing the person's wholeness is the encounter in which nursing lives. The person's unpredictability and uniqueness as a human being serve to render nursing diagnoses inadequate, fractional, and inappropriate. Within the process of knowing persons in their wholeness dwells nursing. In the end, it is the expression of one's self-relating with the other that makes nursing live meaningfully as practice.

REFERENCES

Boykin, A., & Schoenhofer, S. (1993). *Nursing as caring: A model for transforming practice.* New York: National League for Nursing Press.

Dean, B. (1998). Reflections on technology: Increasing the science but diminishing the art of nursing? *Accident and Emergency Nursing, 6*(4), 200–206.

Heidegger, M. (1977). *The question concerning technology and other essays.* New York: Harper and Row.

Henrik, W. (1999). The concept of disease: From Newton back to Aristotle. *The Lancet, 354,* supplement, SIV50.

Leininger, M. (1988). Leininger's theory of nursing: Cultural care diversity and universality. *Nursing Science Quarterly, 1,* 152–160.

Locsin, R. (1995). Machine technologies and caring in nursing. *Image: Journal of Nursing Scholarship, 27*(3), 201–203.

Locsin, R. (1997). Knowing the whole person: Revolutionizing nursing practice. *University of Iceland Nursing Research Paper Series, 1* (suppl.), 359–362.

Locsin, R. (1998). Technological competency as an expression of caring in nursing. *Holistic Nursing Practice, 12*(4), 50–56.

Mayeroff, M. (1971). *On caring.* New York: Harper and Row.

Mitchell, G. (1995). Nursing diagnosis: Obstacle to caring ways. In A. Boykin (Ed.), *Power, politics and public policy.* New York: National League for Nursing.

Purnell, M., & Locsin, R. (2000). *Intentionality: Unification in nursing.* Manuscript submitted for publication.

Roach, S. (1984). *Caring: The human mode of being.* Toronto: University of Toronto Faculty of Nursing.

Shragg, T. (1995, June). Where's the patient in the "industrial model" of care? *The American Nurse, 5,* 7.

Watson, J. (1985). *Nursing: The philosophy and science of caring.* Boulder: Colorado Associated University Press.

Part I

Foundational Concepts of
Technology, Caring, and Nursing

Chapter 1

A Framework for Caring in a Technologically Dependent Nursing Practice Environment

Savina O. Schoenhofer

INTRODUCTION

The practice of twenty-first-century nursing is conducted in environments that rely on complex biomedical machine technology, practice environments that differ vastly from those of an earlier era. The core of nursing, the basic service of nursing, however, has not changed. Caring continues to be the most essential and the most direct expression of nursing service. Nurses now face the challenge of creating an environment of personal care in the context of highly sophisticated, although impersonal, health care technology. This challenge is captured in the poetic expression of one nurse who voiced her own frustration through that reflected on the face of her patient.

Intensive Care

Did you see nurse that you can know me—
The part that is me, my mind and soul is in my eyes
These tubes that are everywhere—that is not me.
The one in my throat is the worst of all—
Now my whole being, the essence of me I
must reflect
through my hands but they are tied down,
movements
of my head but did you realize that
uncomfortable for me
or through my eyes and you do not notice them—
except once today during my bath.
You speak to me and look at the tubes—

Don't you know my thoughts are all over my face
Don't you realize your thoughts are on your face—
In your touch and your tone of voice.
I wrote a request on paper and you said "I'll take care
of it for you" ... your tone said "Why can't this
woman do anything for herself?"
You positioned your hand to count my pulse but I
Can't say you touched me—you wouldn't hold my hand that I may touch you.
You walked in for the first time today with a grin
on your face but your mouth is now tight and
you grimaced a lot as you bathed me.
Don't you see nurse that you can know me—I'm not
a chart or tubes of medication, monitors or all
the other things you look at so intensely—I'm
more than that I'm scared—just look in my eyes.

                                                      Sheila Carr (1991)

The patient's plea, "Don't you see nurse that you can know me," is the universal call for nursing, whatever the setting. Helping nurses hear and answer patients' calls for being known and thus cared for as persons is the focus of this entire volume. The purpose of this chapter is to present fundamental conceptualizations of caring in nursing that can enrich and expand caring consciousness in high-technology environments.

SELECTED FOUNDATIONAL PERSPECTIVES OF CARING IN NURSING

Roach's (1987) philosophical treatise on the human act of caring in nursing and other health professions posits that caring is "the human mode of being" (p. 46). The human act that is caring is the recognition of the intrinsic value of each person and the response to that value. To be human *is* to be caring. Although the capacity to care is innately human, this capacity may lie dormant (Roach, 1987). Human action that does not convey a recognition of the intrinsic value of person is often described as "inhuman." As exemplified in the poem, persons cry out for the caring nurturance of nursing and nurses. Roach's emphasis on caring as *act* is particularly relevant to a practiced discipline such as nursing. Caring is not merely warm feelings or positive regard, but the outward expression or communication of those feelings and sense of regard through a myriad of uniquely creative actions. The patient in "Intensive Care" is calling for an act of recognition; the nurse's failure is a failure to act in recognition of the intrinsic value of the patient: "You wouldn't hold my hand that I may touch you."

In Watson's (1985) theory of human care transactions, caring is described as the moral ideal of nursing. Caring as a process is a reciprocal "I–thou" (Buber, 1937); the embodiment of a commitment to protect, enhance, and preserve human dignity. Again we see that caring is viewed not solely as intention, but as enactment of that intention. Caring preserves a common sense of humanity, as the humanity of one is reflected in the other. When the communication of transpersonal caring is missing in a nursing interaction, both parties are at risk for losing their own sense of being human. The nurse-poet recognizes moments of encounter, as well as lost opportunities to live the moral ideal of caring as she hears the patient say: "my eyes . . . you do not notice them—except once today during my bath."

Parse (1981) defines the ontology of caring as "risking being with someone toward a moment of joy" (p. 130). Caring is the act that expresses true presence and creates a sense of connectedness that brings joy to both the nurse and the one nursed. The joylessness nurses sometimes experience in their work may be the echo of isolation brought on by the reluctance to risk true presence with their patients. The joyful renewal that might be possible through connectedness is foreclosed, and depression and detachment become the norm: "Don't you realize your thoughts are on your face, in your touch and your tone of voice."

Leininger (1988), a nurse-anthropologist, found in her cross-cultural studies that caring is essential for human survival, growth, and development. Leininger's view of caring as act is in accord with other nursing scholars. What counts as care in Leininger's (1988) theoretical view depends on an intracultural understanding of meanings, symbols, and patterns that are expressed through culture care and nursing actions. The intensive care nurse and patient in the poem appear to be functioning in a bicultural human environment rather than one which is transcultural. Transcultural nursing, in which the nurse facilitates the development of culture-sharing, provides the pathway to human connectedness. The pain voiced in the poem is connected to the lack of shared cultural value of meanings, symbols, and patterns of being and acting. The nurse seems to have become enculturated in the impersonal, technologized environment, taking that culture as the ground of meaning, symbols, and patterns, while the patient's world is overlooked: "I'm not a chart or tubes of medication, monitors or all the other things you look at so intensely . . ."

Erikkson (1994) asserts that "true caring is not a form of behavior, not a feeling or a state, it is a being" (p. 11). Caring communion, an unselfish relationship with another, is described as the context of nursing, a way of living, the spirit, the source of power and meaning in caring (Eriksson, 1992a, 1994). The "caritas" motive which provides the fundamental impulse to nurse gives rise to expressions of human love and charity in nursing. "Nursing deficiency, not noticing or understanding the patient's desire for confirmation, can be a sign of lack of courage, lack of compassion, lack of ability to interpret the patient's signals and/or insufficient knowledge of existential/spiritual matters" (Fagerstrom, Erikkson, & Engberg, 1998, p. 984). The nurse-poet does not tell us whether the nursing deficiency described in "Intensive Care" is actual or potential. The power of the poem lies in each nurse's joint recognition of the possibility of personal nursing deficiency and commitment to the caritas motive. The closing plea is one that the nurse as well as the patient may make: "I'm scared—just look in my eyes."

NURSING AS CARING: AN INTEGRATING MODEL

The general theory of Nursing As Caring (Boykin & Schoenhofer, 1993) is offered as a model for integrating nursing philosophical underpinnings of caring, a model that serves as a guide to the caring practice of nursing in situations of complex technological support. After a brief overview of Nursing as Caring, the remainder of this chapter will illustrate the use of the theory to guide practice. The values and concepts of Nursing As Caring will be applied to a transformation of the situation described in the poem "Intensive Care," anticipating that readers can then transfer insights they have gained to their own practice experience in technology-laden settings.

The focus, the aim, the "raison d'être" of nursing from the perspective of Nursing As Caring is to "nurture persons living caring and growing in caring" (Boykin & Schoenhofer, 1993, p. 21). The fundamental assumption underlying this view is that persons *are* caring by virtue of their humanness. The role of the nurse is to:

- enter into the world of the nursed in order to [know person as living caring uniquely] in the moment with personal aspirations for growing in caring and
- to recognize, acknowledge, support, and celebrate the nursed as caring person, thus enhancing the process of personhood, a way of living grounded in caring.

Caring, as it is uniquely expressed through the human service of nursing, may be described as "the intentional and authentic presence of the nurse with another who is recognized as person living caring and growing in caring" (Boykin & Schoenhofer, 1993, p. 25). To truly nurse is to *value this* person in *this* moment, to form the committed *intention* to care and to *communicate* that caring effectively to the nursed. The effective communication of caring requires that each nursing situation be encountered in its uniqueness with immediacy and presence. Nurse caring in high-technology settings is grounded in two fundamental principles: intentionality and knowing.

Like caring, intentionality is much more than diffuse "well-meaning."

Intentionality is the act of forming an intent, joining value, will, and action in a congruent, personal expression and communication. The value that underlies the intent of nursing is conceptualized in the nurse's understanding of the core meaning of nursing. From the perspective of Nursing As Caring, the underlying value is stated in the focus of nursing, "nurturing persons living caring and growing in caring." This understanding of the essential nature of nursing provides the nurse with the wellspring and guiding mission of practice. Nurses whose practice incorporates the use of cognitive and/or mechanical technology understands that when technologies are used for nursing purposes, those uses must be intentional expressions of caring.

Mayeroff (1972) provides a language that can help nurses live their commitment to nursing as a personal mode of living caring values and nurturing others as caring persons. The ingredients of caring proposed by Mayeroff (1972) include: knowing, alternating rhythms, patience, honesty, trust, humility, hope, and courage. Understanding the caring ingredient of knowing is enhanced by Carper's (1979) fundamental patterns of knowing in nursing: personal knowing, ethical knowing, empirical knowing, and esthetic knowing. White (1995) suggested the addition of a fifth pattern, sociopolitical knowing. Munhall (1993) enlarges the connection between knowing and humility in her discussion of "unknowing" as an important pattern.

As stated earlier, caring in nursing is not merely a positive feeling but requires knowledge and understanding for effective action. The poem "Intensive Care" begins and ends with a plea for knowing, both personal knowing and esthetic knowing. Personal knowing as a nursing expression of care involves direct experience, presence, entering into the world of the other with the intention of caring. The patient is calling to be known as person, unique and worthwhile in his/her own right; the nurse gives little evidence of involved presence or personal availability and thus a basic call for nursing goes unanswered. Ethical knowing involves knowing what action is right in a given situation. The nurse in this situation may have known what was right in a technological sense but appears to be unaware of the necessity to know the person she is attempting to nurse as an integral aspect of ethical practice. Empirical knowing, again, may be present in terms of technology; however, a multitude of observational data regarding the patient's desire to be known as person goes unrecognized or ignored. Esthetic knowing comes through appreciating and creating, and involves a deep understanding of the whole picture. It is through esthetic knowing that nurses gain a sustaining sense of well-being from their personal involvement with those they nurse. A nurse who finds him/herself in an impersonal, detached stance toward the patient is one who misses out on the mutual benefits of appreciation and creative expression that is the richness of nursing practice. The nurse depicted in the poem has failed to comprehend the sociopolitical aspects of the situation, the social nature of nursing, and the political ramifications of a role status differential between the nurse on whose turf the practice occurs and the patient whose vulnerability is exquisitely portrayed. Unknowing is a crucial first step to coming to know—the nurse who assumes that one intensive care patient situation is like all the rest is not open to offering true presence and the "nursing care" given is cold, impersonal, and mutually unsatisfying.

This author trusts that the reader is a caring nurse who is living a commitment to growing in personal and professional caring. Therefore, it is not sufficient to merely critique the nursing deficiency illustrated in the poem; it is also necessary to suggest possible avenues leading to the actualization of the caritas motive. Taking for granted the nurse's commitment to care, how might that intention be effectively translated into communicated action?

The ingredient of alternating rhythms means moving back and forth between the microscopic view (example: attention to the proper functioning of machine technologies) and the macroscopic view (example: attention to the person on whose behalf the technologies are being employed). Eye contact facilitates personal connectedness, "my whole being, the essence of me I must reflect . . . through my eyes and you do not notice them," as does listening and language, "you speak to me and look at the tubes" (Erikkson, 1992a). Nurses who are expert at communicating caring effectively in high-technology settings "go to the patient through the technology," not stopping with attending to tubes and monitors, but first connecting with the patient through authentic presence and then attending to technology as an intentional way of caring for the person. In expert nurses, esthetic knowing enables an almost simultaneous perception of both microscopic and macroscopic views. As nurses, we know "person first" is the correct order of things—how do we allow ourselves to engage only with the technology? Perhaps we fear (mis)reading in the patient's eyes an impossible expectation that says "save me," when the patient is really saying, "save me if you can but above all, be with me." Perhaps we are pressed for time in understaffed, overburdened employment situations, thinking "there is no time to care." A nurse's commitment to transcend these barriers and respond to the person as person requires courage, the courage to become vulnerable. Also required is trust, the confidence that our presence, our "being there," is truly a valuable way of caring in any situation. Erikkson (1992b) found, in her study of the meaning and structure of caring communion to nurses and patients, that "Time as a quantity is of no great significance, but the experience of sharing time is important" (p. 92).

Alternating rhythms and the humility of unknowing open the nurse to the realization that the patient has an entire life outside of the intensive care unit, a life whose meanings, symbols, and patterns are very different from those of the hospital. Entering into the world of the other requires discovering and valuing persons in the context of their own lives. When patients enter a health care setting, they are bombarded with messages that they are in a new and sometimes alien culture and generally attempt to respect the meanings, symbols, and patterns of that culture. The caring nurse demonstrates humility in relinquishing cultural domination and seeks to know the other *within* the context of the other's life, and thus is able to promote culture-sharing. With culture-sharing, patients are enabled to make choices that maximize their use of the resources of the health care setting while preserving their own integrity and dignity. How might the nurse promote culture-sharing? The answer lies in living the commitment to coming to know the other as caring person, modifying the environment to the extent possible, and interpreting the culture of the setting to the patient while also interpreting the patient's context to other health care personnel. These actions can help insure that the patient knows s/he is truly valued as the caring person s/he is and is striving to become. Promoting a transcultural environment for nursing requires courage, without which the moments of joy possible in a caring nursing relationship may not be realized.

Communicating authentic presence through touch calls for courage, "you positioned your hand to count my pulse but I can't say you touched me." How does the nurse summon the courage to offer "nothing" but self? Humility as an ingredient of caring strengthens the resolve to care. Hope, an awareness of the moment alive with possibilities, can bring the nurse and nursed into caring communion. Hope encourages the nurse to realize that the gift of self in a transpersonal caring moment awakens self-healing possibilities in the patient and in the nurse as well.

Acknowledging, supporting, and celebrating the nursed as caring person calls for the caring ingredients of patience and honesty. The nurse cares for self by cultivating the patience required to come to know another and to learn new patterns of effectively communicating caring, especially in familiar situations. Honesty as an ingredient of caring leads the nurse to reflect on current patterns of caring and evaluate their effectiveness, "your tone said 'why can't this woman do anything for herself?' " Trust and hope are required if we, as nurses, are to transcend a socially sanctioned focus on troublesome characteristics of patients in order to discover the uniquely personal ways of caring that the patient is expressing. For example, the vulnerability and neediness expressed by the patient, "I'm scared—just look in my eyes," ought to be understood as expressions of caring, requiring honesty, courage, trust, and hope. The nurse celebrates the nursed, responding by valuing the patient's gifts of honesty, trust, and hope and offering the comfort and security of presence and connectedness.

All the ingredients of caring and patterns of knowing are needed as the nurse searches for ways of supporting and celebrating the nursed as caring person. The practice of nursing offers rich opportunities for appreciating and creating and thus contributing to the enhanced personhood of the nursed as well as the nurse, "don't you see nurse that you can know me." As the nurse becomes more skilled in knowing the nursed as caring person, s/he nurtures the other while growing in the spirit of caring that is nursing.

Another poem, "I Care for Him," offers an evocative counterpoint to "Intensive Care," communicating in positive terms what the author of "Intensive Care" advocated by showing the impact on the patient of nursing that did not live up to the moral ideal of caring. "I Care for Him" suggests concepts of caring from the nursing literature and portrays the struggles and satisfaction one nurse experiences through living his intentional commitment to the values and principles of Nursing As Caring.

I Care for Him

My hands are moist,
My heart is quick,
My nerves are taut,
He's in the next room,
I care for him.

The room is tense,
It's anger-filled,
The air seems thick,
I'm with him now,
I care for him.

Time goes slowly by,
As our fears subside,
I can sense his calm,
He softens now,
I care for him.

His eyes meet mine,
Unable to speak,
I feel his trust,
I open my heart,
I care for him.

It's time to leave.
Our bond is made,
Unspoken thoughts,
But understood,
I care for him!

James M. Collins (1993)

REFERENCES

Boykin, A., & Schoenhofer, S. (1991). Caring in nursing: Analysis of extant theory. *Nursing Science Quarterly, 3*, 149–155.

Boykin, A., & Schoenhofer, S. (1993). *Nursing as caring: A model for transforming practice.* New York: National League for Nursing.

Buber, M. (1937). *I and thou.* New York: Scribner.

Carper, B. (1978). Fundamental patterns of knowing in nursing. *Advances in Nursing Science, 1*(1), 13–23.

Carr, S. (1991). Intensive care. *Nightingale Songs, 2*(1). http://www.fau.edu/divdept/nursing/ngsongs/Vol2num1.htm.

Collins, J. (1993). I care for him. *Nightingale Songs, 2*(4). http://www.fau.edu/divdept/nursing/ngsongs/Vol2num4.htm.

Erikkson, K. (1992a). Nursing: The caring practice "being there." In D. A. Gaut (Ed.), *The presence of caring in nursing* (pp. 201–210). New York: National League for Nursing.

Erikkson, K. (1992b). Different forms of caring communion. *Nursing Science Quarterly, 5*, 93.

Erikkson, K. (1994). Theories of caring as health. In D. A. Gaut & A. Boykin (Eds.), *Caring as health: Renewal as hope.* New York: National League for Nursing.

Fagerstrom, L., Eriksson, K., & Engberg, I. B. (1998). The patient's perceived caring needs as a message of suffering. *Journal of Advanced Nursing, 28*, 978–987.

Leininger, M. (1988). Leininger's theory of nursing: Culture care diversity and universality. *Nursing Science Quarterly, 2*(4), 11–20.

Mayeroff, M. (1972). *On caring.* New York: HarperPerennial.

Munhall, P. L. (1993). "Unknowing": Toward another pattern of knowing in nursing. *Nursing Outlook, 41*, 125–128.

Parse, R. R. (1981). Caring from a human science perspective. In M. Leininger (Ed.), *Caring, an essential human need: Proceedings of three National Caring Conferences* (pp. 129–132). Thorofare, NJ: C. B. Slack.

Roach, S. (1987). *The human act of caring.* Ottawa: Canadian Hospital Association.

Watson, J. (1985). *Nursing: Human science and human care, a theory of nursing.* Norwalk, CT: Appleton-Century-Crofts.

White, J. (1995). Patterns of knowing: Review, critique and update. *Advances in Nursing Science, 17*(4), 73–86.

Chapter 2

Technology and Historical Inquiry in Nursing

Alan Barnard and Angela Cushing

INTRODUCTION

This chapter introduces important historical trends that have influenced
the development of technology within the context of nursing. It highlights the need for ongoing research and scholarship that focuses on
technology as a leit motif and examines its implications for the practice
and theory of nursing. Discussion contextualizes the relationship between nursing and technology prior to the eighteenth century and highlights trends that have occurred in the contemporary health care sector.
The necessity of understanding technology as a phenomenon crucial to
the development of nursing knowledge is presented through inquiry into
the significance of hospitals, practice change, and the roles and responsibilities of nurses. It is argued that in the interest of the ongoing quest
within nursing for a broader and deeper knowledge base that brings
greater understanding, nurses need to focus critical attention on the history of technology and nursing.

Technology is a complex interrelationship between numerous influential characteristics that include machinery, equipment, tools, utensils,
automata, apparatus, structures, clothes and utilities (technical objects),
people, organizations, science, culture, gender, values, and politics, based
on the goals of efficiency and logical order. Technology is significant to
nurses and society. It has transformed the workplace, not only in terms
of the machinery and equipment used, but how and why nurses use
them. Because of these transformations, an ideological awareness is required in which we are all reeducated about the relationship between
technology and gender, politics, national economic survival, and the cul-

ture of individual societies and groups (Barnard, 1999b, 2000b; Dunphy, 1985; Fairman & D'Antonio 1999).

In contemporary health care, the practices of many occupational groups (such as nurses) have been defined according to bureaucratic, economic, and behavioral criteria, and they have been transformed into subspecialties. Despite these changes to the organization of nurses and most forms of employment, there has been failure by employers, governments, unions, educators, employees, and managers to stress the importance of these transformations and to highlight their influential effects upon the workplace. Winner (1977) argues that "although people are aware of their changing world and the development of new organizational systems, their awareness is at the level of intuition and passivity and their understanding is rarely linked to the development of technology" (p. 207).

We live with the costs and do not make the connections to their origins. Many nurse historians, academics, clinicians, and critics do not examine adequately the significance and meaning of technology. For example, there is limited knowledge of the historical evolution of nursing technology or the reasons why certain technical objects have become important to nursing practice. Inadequate explanation of the experience of technology and simplistic explanation of the phenomenon have continued to restrict the development of nursing. Adequate understanding of nursing will emerge only when nurses recognize technology as influential in the organization of human labor and fundamental to its moral, political, and professional goals (Barnard, 1997; Donahue, 1985; Harding, 1980). An informed explanation of the historical and contemporary importance of technology to nursing is needed because current practices contribute to ineffective interactions with patients and nature. They support access to the social benefits of technological change by privileged groups. There has been a failure to make technology appropriately visible in health care apart from encouragement for nurses to engage in further instrumental involvement. The invisibility is so marked that it has been claimed that anyone attempting to understand nursing and technology is standing on shifting ground (Sandelowski, 1999).

NURSING AND TECHNOLOGY PRIOR TO THE EIGHTEENTH CENTURY

Nurses have always used tools and techniques in meaningful ways to achieve valued ends. Prior to this century, nursing was essentially as it had been throughout history, a craft practiced by individuals of whom the majority were women. They gained experience in caregiving from religious and secular orders or through families. Knowledge and skills developed by trial and error and were passed on, generation by generation, through an oral culture. Nursing practice relied upon rule of thumb, experience, and faith, and was isolated to groups of individuals and geographic areas. Skills and beliefs included magical and aesthetic components that were associated with moral and psychic life. Appropriately trusted and well-intentioned individuals effected treatment that could not be translated into scientific language or rationale. Nurses relied less on scientific knowledge than on a personal and intuitive understanding developed and refined through practice (Abel-Smith, 1960; Baly, 1995; Barnard, 1996; Dock & Stewart, 1925; Reverby, 1987).

Technology did not present Western society with many challenges associated with social adaptation, morality, or ethics, prior to the beginning of the third industrial revolution. The third industrial revolution is generally argued to be associated with advances in commerce and industry in the eighteenth century. Societal changes from this revolution have been both qualitative and quantitative, and emerge particularly from advances in science and technology. The period marked a change from agrarian and handicraft economies to economies dominated by industry and machine manufacture. Landes (1969, p. 1) distinguished the period as noteworthy for three spheres of change: (1) mechanical devices began to replace human skills; (2) non-human power (steam followed by fossil fuel and atomic energy) dominated human strength; and (3) raw materials increased leading to rapid developments in metallurgical and chemical industries. Prior to this period, the evolution of technology was slow and expertise was based on the know-how of a person who used an expert eye and was distinguishable for his or her particular style and precision. The slow evolution meant that technical advance rarely threatened social equilibrium and was assimilated into society (Ellul, 1964; Kranzberg & Pursell, 1967; Mumford, 1934).

TECHNOLOGY AND THE MODERN ERA

The rapid growth of scientific and technological knowledge in Western society since the eighteenth century has produced enormous changes in nursing and health care. Science and technology have influenced many facets of nursing practice, awareness, and experience. In addition, there have been numerous social challenges associated particularly with adapting precepts to a rapidly changing social milieu, the exploitation of people, the division of classes, and increases in poverty. However, like society, many nurses have encouraged an adoration of technological progress and have both welcomed and encouraged continued involvement with technological change (Barnard, 1996, 1999a; Sandelowski, 1997). In fact, Cooper (1993, p. 25) goes so far as to assert that the process of technological advancement has grown to an extent that the environments of nursing practice are no longer defined by human caring but by machine technology.

Despite the significance of technology to the experience of nurses, the phenomenon has been examined inadequately within the context of both nursing practice and nursing's quest for knowledge. There is limited historical awareness of the influence of technology or understanding of the philosophical and social significance of its emergence (Allan & Hall, 1988; Barnard, 1996, 2000a, 2000b; Fairman, 1996; Fairman & Lynaugh, 1998; Reverby, 1987; Sandelowski, 1996; Walters, 1995). Christman (1970, p. 13) noted that the history of nursing has been one in which nurses have concentrated on looking inward and viewing the remainder of the world as hostile. Folta (1973) builds on the assertion and argues that "since the advent of modern science and technology, health care professionals have dealt with philosophical problems by ignoring them" (p. 35).

Historical accounts of nursing emphasize achievements in professional standing, administrative acumen, educational development, and purposeful unity. While these achievements are of note, their emphases have overridden serious review of the origin and impact of political, economic, and social trends. Historical influences important to the development of nursing have not been given credence, and it has become difficult to consider nursing in a more precise way (Baly, 1986; Cushing, 1994; Maggs, 1983). For example, historical texts, nursing literature, and manuals of nursing practice have rarely critiqued the social and professional impact of technology. Kranzberg and Pursell (1967) claimed three decades ago that these types of challenges are common historical and sociological issues. Individuals and occupational groups continue to ignore both the social outcomes of technological development and the way individuals think about technology. Analysis of technology is restricted generally to opinion and description of internal history (e.g., machinery, periods of technological advance, industrial revolutions). The outcomes of technology such as the evolution of the moral and ethical debate, the experience of technology, and its impact upon disciplines, are absent.

Early nursing texts express utopian ideas about nursing, society, and the impact of technology (Abel-Smith, 1960; Jamieson, 1966; Roberts, 1954; Shryock, 1959). The history and experience of technological development is not addressed and technology is conceived uncritically as an instrumental phenomenon that advances the profession. While advancement may or may not be true, the lack of historical perspicacity and consequent absence of historical interpretation in relation to the role of technology in the context of nursing has other implications related to nursing's knowledge quest. First, the lack of historical insight has meant that nursing literature has come to be dominated by an embryonic understanding of the place of technology in the historical development of nursing knowledge. Second, the absence of critique has not encouraged reflection on accepted and future practices. For example, Hiraki (1992) demonstrated, through an examination of four introductory nursing textbooks, that little is known about the social, ideological, and political issues that influence textbook development. Dominant themes found in nursing texts are rationality of language, a propensity to overemphasize the pseudo-scientific approach called the nursing process, and instrumentalism. Hiraki (1992) argued that "the world of the textbook discloses how nurses interpret their professional autonomy and how normative structures inform what constitutes authority and responsibility in research, education and practice. [In particular] . . . the language and rationality of all four textbooks limit the possibility of self-critique and reflection" (p. 11).

HOSPITALS AND NURSING

An important factor in understanding the relationship between technology and the history of nursing is the hospital. Few institutions have undergone such rapid and radical change as hospitals have throughout this century. Hospitals have evolved from being institutions responsible for the care of the destitute to a visible embodiment of the health care sector and corporate development. Rapid developments in science and technology and the expansion of institutionalized medicine have meant that hospitals have become responsible for the provision and development of medical investigation, treatment, and research. Centralized resources, specialist staff, and technique have evolved to become features of hospitals. Diagnosis, treatment, and research into acute illnesses have become their primary purposes and have prevailed over issues of religious and moral concern (Maggs, 1983; Reiser, 1978; Reverby, 1987).

Although credit is awarded to nursing schools for their role in stimulating the emergence of nursing as an occupation in this century, equal emphasis must be awarded to the evolution of the hospital. According to numerous authors, the emergence of nursing as an occupation has come from increases in work demands and opportunities within hospitals, rather than any specific political coup or planned development for nursing (Baly, 1986; Fairman & D'Antonio, 1999; Fairman & Lynaugh, 1998; Maggs, 1983; Reverby, 1987). Despite nurse education advancements, and the influence of nurses in improving treatment conditions within hospitals through the introduction of major reforms to physical environments and the practices of both themselves and doctors, nursing has remained a subservient occupation whose major role has been to provide cheap labor for the hospital sector.

Nurses continue to be controlled often by hospital administrators and medicine in an institutionalized health care sector where the central concern is efficiency and the advancement of medical science and technology. To this day, nurses continue to struggle for power and recognition, and they seek to produce good practitioners for clinical environments where technical performance is highly prized.

THE DEPUTIZATION OF NURSING

With the development of the hospital in this century, nurses have accepted new roles and responsibilities that have originated from the introduction of new technologies to nursing practice and the reassignment of duties from medicine and administrators. The reassignment of roles and responsibilities is a process that can be defined as deputization. The word "deputization" means: depute (di pyut'); to appoint to do one's work or to act in one's place; delegate (Barnhart & Barnhart, 1994, p. 562).

Deputization is an ongoing process in nursing and is characterized by the acceptance of various technical and administrative roles and responsibilities from other health care providers who retain a supervisory capacity and some professional responsibility (i.e., decision making and governorship). Dock and Stewart (1925) identified the beginning of the process early this century:

Many nurses specialize in various forms of therapeutics, X-ray and electrical treatment, hydrotherapy, massage, etc. Others assist in the new field of laboratory work in the study of metabolism. There is, also, a tendency to give to the nurse some of the hospital duties formerly assigned to the intern, as, the giving of anesthetics, keeping of records, and other clinical ward work. (p. 304)

Notwithstanding, as a result of the reassignment of duties and a redefining of clinical roles and responsibilities, nurses have discerned a sense of involvement with science and technology in a technologically dominated health care sector that relies increasingly on nurses to fulfill an instrumental role in the provision of health care. Their increasing inclusion in the use of machinery and equipment is often interpreted by nurses as a demonstration of their role in the success of science and technology, and their skills are a visible embodiment of technological development (Cooper, 1993; Gordon, 1992; McClure, 1991).

Despite the ongoing evolution of deputization and the subsequent expectation that nurses will continue to accept expanded roles and responsibilities, issues related to technology have rarely been stated in terms of changes to nursing goals, technological dominance, or alterations in nursing practice (Sanford, 1967). Nurses have been interested less in questioning the prestige and power of science and technology than in embellishing their development. Nurses have displayed no resistance to assuming responsibility for all manner of tasks and knowledge associated with the emergence of technology, and have subsequently absorbed roles and responsibilities into their professional experience and structure (Castledine, 1995; Donahue, 1985; Walker, 1970). As a consequence, medicine has delegated time-consuming and repetitious tasks to nurses; tasks associated with routine treatment, monitoring, observation, and investigation (Brown, 1992; Fairman & Lynaugh, 1998; Reverby, 1987).

Reiser (1978) observed that delegation of responsibility is often seen as proper and necessary in carrying out work on a large scale because the doctor can "determine whether the work was conducted in the proper manner, and he [sic] accepted responsibility for it. This was the case when the physician delegated his [sic] duties to the resident staff of the hospital, the director of laboratory to his [sic] staff, or the practitioner to his [sic] nurse" (p. 172).

As a consequence of these changes, nurses have reached a point in their development where they need to examine nursing practice. Even though delegation has occasionally been to the mutual interdisciplinary benefit of nurses and doctors, it is argued that critical examination of nursing highlights the extent to which doctors, administrators, and nurses have abraded the practice of nursing (Brown, 1992; Donahue, 1985; Fairman & D'Antonio, 1999; Jacox, Pillar, & Redman, 1990; Pellegrino & Thomasma, 1981). Deputization of nursing can be described as extending the goals of medicine, and on many occasions de-emphasizing the roles of nursing, particularly the fundamental care of the person (e.g., hygiene). Nursing can be characterized as being consumed by both other health care providers and nurses who seek professional respect as a result of the use of technical objects, diagnostic roles, and treatment responsibility. Briggs (1991) agrees with this assessment and suggests that experience and evidence is demonstrating, for example, that because of technology the "technical skills associated with nursing a patient just after an operation were [are] far more prestigious than the nursing skills involved in caring for the longer term patients" (p. 26).

Although nobody would argue against the need for nursing to be responsive to the demands of the health care sector, limited knowledge is available to acknowledge or refute arguments concerning the extent, effect, and experience of technology. Nurses are responsible for an increasingly machinery-oriented health care system that is significant for its administrative and bureaucratic structures. Nurses in all specialties of practice are required to care for their patients, develop technical knowledge and skills, and respond to the requirements of the health care system. They are required to not only manipulate machinery and interpret the world around them, but take on increasingly varied and complex roles and responsibilities associated with the emergence of technology (Allan & Hall, 1988; Barnard, 1997, 1999b; Wichowski & Kubsch, 1995). The history, meaning, and implications of technology for practice and nursing knowledge will not be understood fully without due attention to further research, scholarship, and theoretical development.

CONCLUDING REMARKS

Nurses need to make choices in their commitment to technology and recognize the importance of becoming more aware, and appropriately critical of, the phenomenon. If nursing practice is influenced directly by the values of society and groups (Wilkinson, 1992), more needs to be done to understand the relationship between technology and the history of nursing. In particular, historical research and scholarship that seek to illuminate the relationship between technology and politics, gender, and economic development, as well as those processes central to the inclusion of nurses in the development of technological health care, are central. Further to this, analysis of inventions and developments that have arisen directly from nursing will be an advantage to understanding technology as an important phenomenon in the history of nursing. This chapter has offered an introductory exploration of important trends related to technology and nursing history. It contributes to the complex and burgeoning interest of nurses who are attempting to bring understanding to the importance of technology.

REFERENCES

Abel-Smith, B. (1960). *A history of the nursing profession*. London: Heinemann.

Allan, J. D., & Hall, B. A. (1988). Challenging the focus on technology: A critique of the medical model in a changing health care system. *Advances in Nursing Science, 10*(3), 22–34.

Baly, M. (1986). *Florence Nightingale and the nursing legacy*. London: Croom Helm.

Baly, M. (1995). *Nursing and social change* (3rd ed.). London: Routledge.

Barnard, A. (1996). Technology and nursing: An anatomy of definition. *International Journal of Nursing Studies, 33*(4), 433–441.

Barnard, A. (1997). A critical review of the belief that technology is a neutral object and nurses are its master. *Journal of Advanced Nursing, 26*(1), 126–131.

Barnard, A. (1999a). Nursing and the primacy of technological progress. *International Journal of Nursing Studies, 36*, 435–442.

Barnard, A. (1999b). Technology and the Australian nursing experience. In J. Daly, S. Speedy, & D. Jackson (Eds.), *Contexts of nursing: An introduction* (pp. 163–176). Sydney: Maclennan & Petty.

Barnard, A. (2000a). Alteration to will as an experience of technology and nursing. *Journal of Advanced Nursing, 31*(5), 1136–1144.

Barnard, A. (2000b). Towards an understanding of technology and nursing practice. In J. Greenwood (Ed.), *Nursing theory in Australia: Development and application* (2nd ed.) (In Press). Sydney: HarperCollins.

Barnhart, C., & Barnhart, R. (1994). *The World Book Dictionary*. Chicago: Scott Fettzer.

Briggs, D. (1991). Critical care nurses' roles—traditional or expanded/extended. *Intensive Care Nursing, 7,* 223–229.

Brown, J. (1992). Nurses or technicians? The impact of technology on oncology nursing. *Canadian Oncology Nursing Journal, 2*(1), 12–17.

Castledine, G. (1995). Issues for nursing in 1995. *British Journal of Nursing, 4*(1), 45.

Christman, L. (1970). What the future holds for nurses. *Nursing Forum, 9*(1), 13–18.

Cooper, M. C. (1993). The intersection of technology and care in the ICU. *Advances in Nursing Science, 15*(3), 23–32.

Cushing, A. (1994). Historical and epistemological perspectives on research and nursing. *Journal of Advanced Nursing, 20,* 406–411.

Dock, L., & Stewart, I. (1925). *A short history of nursing*. New York: Putnam's.

Donahue, M. (1985). *Nursing: The finest art. An illustrated history*. St. Louis, MO: Mosby.

Dunphy, D. (1985). Technological change and its impact on industrial democracy. *Work and People, 11*(2), 17–20.

Ellul, J. (1964). *The technological society*. New York: Alfred A. Knopf.

Fairman, J. (1996). Response to tools of the trade: Analyzing technology as object in nursing. *Scholarly Inquiry for Nursing Practice: An International Journal, 10*(1), 17–21.

Fairman, J., & D'Antonio, P. (1999). Virtual power: Gendering the nurse-technology relationship. *Nursing Inquiry, 6,* 178–186.

Fairman, J., & Lynaugh, J. E. (1998). *Critical care nursing: A history*. Philadelphia: University of Pennsylvania Press.

Folta, J. (1973). Humanization of services and the use of technology in health care. *The Hong Kong Nursing Journal, 15*(11), 35–39.

Gordon, S. (1992). The importance of being nurses. *Technology Review, 95*(7), 42–51.

Harding, S. (1980). Value laden technologies and the politics of nursing. In S. F. Spicker, & S. Gadow (Eds.), *Nursing: Images and ideals* (pp. 49–75). New York: Springer.

Hiraki, A. (1992). Tradition, rationality, and power in introductory nursing textbooks: A critical hermeneutics study. *Advances in Nursing Science, 14*(3), 1–12.

Jacox, A., Pillar, B., & Redman, B. (1990). A classification of nursing technology. *Nursing Outlook, 38*(2), 81–85.

Jamieson, E. (1966). *Trends in nursing history: Their social international and ethical relationships*. Philadelphia: Saunders.

Kranzberg, M., & Pursell, C. (1967). *Technology in western civilization,* Vol. 2. London: Oxford University Press.

Landes, D. (1969). *The unbound Prometheus: Technological change and industrial development in Western Europe from 1750 to the present*. Cambridge: Cambridge University Press.

Maggs, C. (1983). *The origins of general nursing*. London: Croom Helm.

McClure, M. (1991). Technology—a driving force for change. *Journal of Professional Nursing, 7*(3), 144.

Mumford, L. (1934). *Technics and civilization.* New York: Harcourt Brace.

Pellegrino, E. D., & Thomasma, D. C. (1981). *A philosophical basis of medical practice.* Oxford: Oxford University Press.

Reiser, S. J. (1978). *Medicine and the reign of technology.* Cambridge: Cambridge University Press.

Reverby, S. (1987). *Ordered to care: The dilemma of American nursing, 1850–1945.* Cambridge: Cambridge University Press.

Roberts, M. (1954). *American nursing: History and interpretation.* New York: Macmillan.

Sandelowski, M. (1996). Tools of the trade: Analyzing technology as object in nursing. *Scholarly Inquiry for Nursing Practice: An International Journal, 10*(1), 5–16.

Sandelowski, M. (1997). (Ir)Reconcilable differences? The debate concerning nursing and technology. *Image: Journal of Nursing Scholarship, 29*(2), 169–174.

Sandelowski, M. (1999). Nursing, technology and the millennium. *Nursing Inquiry, 6,* 145.

Sanford, C. (1967). Technology and culture at the end of the nineteenth century: The will to power press. In M. Kranzberg & C. Pursell (Eds.), *Technology in western civilization,* Vol. 2 (pp. 726–740). London: Oxford University Press.

Shryock, R. (1959). *The history of nursing: An interpretation of the social and medical factors involved.* Philadelphia: W. B. Saunders.

Walker, D. (1970). Our challenging world. *Nursing Forum, 9*(4), 328–339.

Walters, A. J. (1995). Technology and the lifeworld of critical care nursing. *Journal of Advanced Nursing, 22,* 338–346.

Wichowski, H. C., & Kubsch, S. (1995). How nurses react to and cope with uncertainty of familiar technology: Validation for continuing education. *The Journal of Continuing Education in Nursing, 26*(4), 174–178.

Wilkinson, P. (1992). The influence of high technology care on patients, their relatives and nurses. *Intensive and Critical Care Nursing, 8*(4), 194–198.

Winner, L. (1977). *Autonomous technology.* Cambridge, MA: MIT Press.

Chapter 3

Pictures of Paradox: Technology, Nursing, and Human Science

Gail J. Mitchell

INTRODUCTION

There is no question that technology makes important contributions to the efficacy, efficiency, and quality of health care, and to quality of life in general. The tools and machines of everyday living provide a constant reminder of the ingenuity of humankind. Scientists are pushing frontiers of space-dwelling and genetic cloning, while computers enable people to relate on a global scale. Innovations in health care, such as topical applications of medication and home dialysis, will increasingly support persons in their self-care activities; and the possibility of launching computer chips into human blood vessels for the purposes of altering cellular processes or genetic codes stretches one's imagination about the future prevention, diagnosis, and treatment of disease. The potential opportunities accompanying technological advances are indeed wondrous, and, at times, perplexing.

However, the technological advances also raise probing questions about boundaries and whether or not people should invent tools and techniques just because they can be invented (Barger-Lux & Heaney, 1986; Crawshaw, 1983). Boundaries and questions of *should* also hold relevance for nurses and their understanding of the role of technology in nursing. The purposes of this chapter are to explore the role of technology in nursing and to consider how the focus on technology has reinforced the thinking and making of the dominant culture of mechanistic nursing.

Mechanistic nursing in this chapter refers to the teaching nurses have received about how to assess, diagnose, and manage human beings. The term refers to the way human beings are conceptualized in component parts, such as bio-psycho-social, body-mind-spirit, and emotional-physical-spiritual. Mechanistic thinking may be necessary to help nurses to know how to manage technology, but it will not help nurses create meaningful partnerships with persons who happen to be patients. The literature supports the belief that people who enter health care systems want to be listened to, supported, respected, and involved as equals in their care (Deegan, 1993; Gerteis et al., 1993; Mitchell & Lawton, 2000; Young-Mason, 1997).

It is proposed here that mechanistic thinking hinders nurses' efforts to practice in ways that uphold nursing's commitment to honor, care, respect, and help. Assessment, judgment, and control have become the hallmarks of the nursing process—and thus, in many instances, of the nurse–person relationship. That most nurses focus on assessing, judging, and managing patients is true, despite the efforts of some nurses to highlight the need for caring, empathy, and touch. It is my experience that the boundaries of mechanism have extended into the nurse–person process in ways that go far beyond concerns about hard and soft technologies. The position here is consistent with others who believe that technology is as much about assumptions, beliefs, and intentions as it is about tools and applications (Barger-Lux & Heaney, 1986; Bernardo, 1998; Gadow, 1984; Kim, 2000; Parse, 1999; Szawarski, 1989).

Gadow (1984) suggested, "The violation of dignity and autonomy that seems to accompany technology is in reality a result not of the role of machines in patient care but of the view of the body as a machine" (p. 65). I believe that the concern is not limited to nurses' focus on the body as a machine, but that many nurses view human life, the lived experience of persons, as mechanistic or machine-like. By this I mean that many nurses believe they can manipulate, manage, change, direct, control, and discharge human beings in ways comparable to how they perform these activities with machines and technology.

From Szawarski's (1989) view, efforts to control others represent an assault against human dignity. Many nurses believe they are responsible for how others think and act, and they make efforts to control people even though history and experience shows that human beings will fiercely resist uninvited controls on their freedoms and rights to choose. Szawarski (1989) suggests resistance to outside control is about one's moral integrity because, "I respect myself when I am able to determine my own behaviour and to act in accordance with my own decisions" (p. 245). The view of life and lived experience as machine-like, and thus controllable, diverts many nurses from their primary mandate: to care for human beings through relationships that enhance health and quality of life from the client's perspective. It will be proposed here that the mechanistic view of human beings is the single greatest threat to pro-

Figure 1
Picture of Paradox

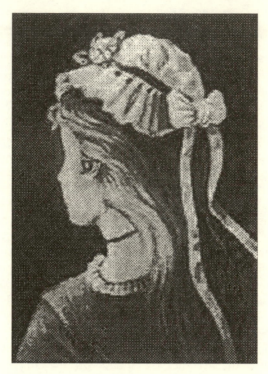

Source: © 1997 IllusionWorks, L.L.C. Reprinted with permission.

fessional nursing and to practices that seek to uphold human dignity, freedom, and quality of life.

PICTURES OF PARADOX AND THE PARADOX OF PARADIGMS

In order to lay the groundwork for what will follow in this chapter, the author offers a description of pictures of paradox to help clarify the complexity of thinking that informs nursing practice and research. Pictures of paradox, common to most people, depict an image that transforms to a completely different image when viewers shift their perspective of what it is they are looking at. Some of the most common images of paradox include a picture of an old woman that is also an image of a young girl's profile (see Figure 1), a duck that is also a rabbit, and a water vase that can also be seen as the profile of two persons facing each other.

When people first look at these pictures of paradox, one image is clearly present while the other is typically absent from view. Two readers may look at the picture of paradox included here, and one may see an old woman while the other sees a young girl's profile. As long as people think they are looking at a single image, the dominant view stays in focus. However, once the other image, also present in the picture, is pointed out, or by chance discovered, viewers can suddenly discern, often with surprise, the second image that comes into view with the same clarity and detail of the first image.

Once persons know that there are two distinct images in the picture, they can intentionally shift their view between the two portraits, seeing in one instant the old woman and in the next the young girl. Of importance to this current exploration into technology, human science, and nursing is the understanding that essential to the experience of the picture of paradox is the viewer's knowledge that the two distinct images coexist simultaneously, and can, when desired, be selected and brought into view. Once two distinct images are viewed, the single image of either is seen with the knowing of the other. What was a simplistic picture of one image becomes a complex picture of paradox with two different, coexisting images. The notion of pictures of paradox will be used here to assist understanding of the complex realities of a discipline struggling to find clarity among the shifting views of scientific paradigms in nursing practice and research. In this examination of scientific paradigms in nursing, one image in Figure 1, it does not matter which, will represent the assumptions and beliefs of the human science paradigm and the other image will represent the mechanistic or technical paradigm of nursing.

THE ORIGINS OF SCIENTIFIC PARADIGMS

The origins of the mechanistic paradigm are primarily attributed to those who worked to discover and control the natural laws that determine human behavior. Allegiance to the methods of Newtonian physics was believed to be the best way to eliminate guesswork, dogma, history, and personal prejudice as science progressed. It was proposed that reason would some day rule and people would be enlightened by truths about humans that could be verified through systematic study and experimentation. Knowledge in the mechanistic paradigm followed the trail of logically deduced conclusions underpinned by principles of control, observation, randomization, and verification through the science of mathematics. According to Berlin (1997), this dominant view of reality has fueled passionate resistance for hundreds of years.

Resistance to the mechanistic paradigm has also been strongly expressed by nurses who claim that there is another paradigm of science that can inform nurses and members of other disciplines who are interested in moving beyond the mechanistic views of human beings (Newman, 1994; Parse, 1981, 1998; Watson, 1995). Nurses writing about nursing as a human science are trying to help others see that there is an opposing paradigm or set of beliefs that can represent a coexisting reality, just like the second image in the picture of paradox.

Human science beliefs have been explicated by various authors in different disciplines (see, for example, Dilthey, 1961, 1976, 1977, 1988; Giorgi, 1970, 1985; Guba & Lincoln, 1990; Parse, 1981, 1987, 1998; Polkinghorne, 1988; Watson, 1985). Mitchell and Cody (1992) presented a synthesis of essential human science beliefs that include the following. First, humans are unitary, irreducible beings who each possess a unique view of the world and who are in continuous interrelationship with their historical, contemporary, and cultural worlds. Second, human experience as lived and as expressed in thinking, feeling, and acting is preeminent, meaning lived experience is the focus for practice and research activities in the human science paradigm. The third essential belief is that humans are intentional and free-willed, always moving on with purpose to new possibilities. This means that in any given situation, people freely choose what things mean, how they will act, and for what they hope and dream. The notions of intentionality and change are linked to the proposed reality that human beings make choices based on their concerns and on what they hope will or will not happen (Parse, 1981, 1998). This is true even when an illness, injury, or other critical event surfaces in day-to-day life.

So, for instance, a single mother may decide not to investigate some episodes of chest pain she is experiencing because she is fearful of leaving her young children; or, a mother may take her baby to an emergency room with complaints that the baby has a slight fever because she knows that if she has to listen to the baby cry for one more hour she might harm the child; or, a father injures himself after working 30 hours without sleep because he wants his children to have opportunities he did not have in life. Human beings make decisions based on their personal experiences, value priorities, concerns, fears, hopes, dreams, and desires, and this fact is rarely acknowledged or valued in health care settings where nurses practice.

Many health care professionals (including some nurses) engage persons, who are living and struggling with their own issues and concerns, with the air of paternalistic judgment that accompanies the mechanistic model. Doctors or nurses might label these people with various disparaging terms and then proceed to tell each of them what they are doing wrong or what they should do in the future. Some nurses might explain to the woman with chest pain that she has to look after herself because what good is she to her children if she ends up in the hospital, or even dead; or, they might tell the young mother with the crying child she should not come to the emergency room for such non-critical issues. It has been my experience that people are viewed as *abusers* of the system if they seek help in an emergency room for things that professionals do not view as important; but could it be that the system is not yet designed to best meet the needs of people?

The biomedical model establishes a judgmental process that labels people as right-wrong, normal-abnormal, realistic-unrealistic, and functional-dysfunctional. Perhaps, more importantly, the mechanistic model encourages the belief that nurses have the right to try to correct others' lives, and many health care professionals expect that others should comply with expert directives. These health directives are sometimes given without full or even partial consideration or regard for the lived experience of the person.

In the mechanistic model, professionals are portrayed as experts who know what is best. But the paternalistic attitude of the mechanistic model is not generally viewed as helpful by patients. Consider the words of Macurdy (1997), who lives with muscular dystrophy.

Far too commonly, a doctor or nurse enters my hospital room and speaks to another professional or to a family member rather than to me. Medical staff have also tried to order for me in restaurants, make requests for me in department stores, and take it upon themselves to reprimand the concierge in my apartment building because the elevator was not working—all in the name of my health care. Such actions are not only corrosive to my self-esteem but undermine my personal interactions and professional integrity by advancing the perception that my needs are so extensive as to render me irrelevant and nearly invisible. (p. 13)

In contrast, nursing actions in the human science tradition are linked to how nurses participate with persons as they experience life, with all the complexity of their personal histories, families, cultures, and unique perspectives. The paradigm of human science requires that nurses, in their thinking and in their actions, honor the unity of lived experience and refrain from dividing persons' experiences into psychological, sociological, cultural, and spiritual problems. Problem lists provide no useful understanding of persons because they depict an outsider's view, an objective interpretation of others' experiences. The focus in the human science paradigm is on honoring persons' experiences and respecting their unique views of life, not on correcting their views and choices. Human science nursing is about giving messages of unconditional regard for others' personal realities in every situation. Any judgment of the person in the nurse–person process would shift the nurse's view from the human to the mechanistic paradigm of practice. This is so because judgment and comparison shift the focus away from the person's experience to what the nurse thinks of the person's experience. The person's lived experience is what it is, a complex unity, a mystery, a process to be respected, not judged. Judgment calls up the alternative image in the picture of paradox and it is, as noted by Macurdy (1997), a way of making the person invisible.

There is no call for judgment in the human science paradigm, because the nurse's goal is not to control how human beings think, but rather to enhance opportunities for persons to discover insights that clarify meanings, options, and choices. Recall the essential belief that human beings are intentional and free-willed. This means that people choose what things mean, what is important, what is worthy of concern, what options are possible, what is desired, and what decisions they will make. People choose when and how they will change. The nurse who holds the human science image in the picture of paradox engages people with the intent to bear witness to their meanings, struggles, and considerations, and there is no intent or desire on the nurse's part to manage or manipulate others' experiences (Parse, 1987, 1998). The human science paradigm directs the nurse to believe that persons are self-directed and self-defining, and therefore people choose how they will change. The opportunity for nurses is to choose ways of participating with people; ways that facilitate others' exploration, discovery, and clarification of hopes and plans for change. Such participation requires respectful dialogue, not assessment; listening, not explaining; accepting, not comparing. The shifting views of mechanistic and human science, of control and freedom, and of lived experience versus objective reality have been hotly debated for hundreds of years.

It is important to note that the discussion here is not about how to make the mechanistic paradigm more humanistic, empathic, or caring. Nurses have already demonstrated how caring and empathy can fit with technology (Jones & Alexander, 1993; Locsin, 1995; McConnell, 1998; Ray, 1987). However, it is proposed here that these authors, despite efforts to sustain values for the whole, unique person, have not yet explicated a substantive and distinct knowledge base that can withstand the overbearing influence of the mechanistic paradigm and its deployment of reductionistic language, judgmental assessment, and edict to manage. The melding of caring and technology does not create a paradoxical knowledge base capable of sustaining human science thinking and acting in the nurse-person process. The absence of human science thinking is evident in nursing practice today, even though most nurses have been taught to be caring, respectful of diverse beliefs, open to individual preferences, and concerned about the whole person—as well as technically competent.

It is not unusual to hear many nurses say that they are too busy to care, too busy to talk to patients/clients, and too busy to listen. Priorities are directed at completing tasks even though patients report that the quality of relationships with nurses has an important and lasting impact on their health experience and quality of life. When talking does happen with clients, it often reflects nurses giving directives and explanations (Deveaux & Babin, 1994, 1996), rather than asking clients open-ended questions. The literature offers examples of how nurses, through their attitudes, words, and actions, can diminish quality and even harm patients and families (see, for example, Baier, 1996; Deegan, 1993; Fisher, 1994; Gerteis et al., 1993; Nagle, 1998; Schroeder, 1998; Young-Mason, 1997). It is suggested here that it is not the matter of time that limits nurses in their relationships with patients, but rather the beliefs and values of the mechanistic paradigm. Mechanistic knowledge cannot direct practice in ways that uphold nurses' intent to connect and make a difference with patients, and this disconnect between paradigm and desired quality of practice diminishes satisfaction for both patient and nurse. Patients' descriptions of their health experiences should inspire all nurses to continue clarifying and thinking about paradigms and how they inform practice.

The picture of paradox described above offers a way for nurses to shift their thinking and acting with persons in light of the contexts and boundaries that define two opposing and sustaining realities. The opposing paradigms provide an essential tension of difference and dissonance that helps nurses recognize and shift between diverging views in the context of moments where nursing practice happens with others. Indeed, the opposing beliefs are essential to hold in one's thinking, just like the images embedded in the picture of paradox. If nurses become comfortable with the notion of pictures of paradox and the process of shifting views, both the mechanistic and human science paradigms can inform practice simultaneously.

The mechanistic paradigm includes knowledge of technology and task, normal physiology and pathophysiology, assessment and cure, prescription and control, intervention and outcome. Within this paradigm, nurses are expected to perform and assist with complex medical procedures. They are expected to learn how to control intricate machines and to understand how the human body changes with disease. Nurses know about chemical and surgical interventions and the potential dangers of these interventions. Nurses are called on to be vigilant in their assessment of subtle changes in bodily function and they carry the formidable responsibility of knowing when to take actions—actions that in many situations save human lives. The knowledge of the mechanistic paradigm informs and guides what nurses do and how they think in many situations, especially in hospital settings. The value of mechanistic (also known as biomedical) knowledge, especially in this age of technology and modern health care, is irrefutable. But, and I cannot emphasize this enough, there is a serious conundrum with the mechanistic paradigm and its related knowledge for guiding nursing activities and for defining nurses' responsibilities to and with human beings.

The conundrum is the human being, the person, who is there in the picture, awaiting discovery as a totally different entity from the mechanistic entities with which it coexists. Many nurses, like other health professionals, do not know about the opposing paradigm of human science as they go about their day-to-day practices within the predominant mechanistic culture. Even though nurses know about caring, empathy, and dignity, they do not have a knowledge base of substance that can sustain the alternative practice of human science. Most professionals relate to only one view of reality; one mechanistic paradigm extended to inform all activities with human beings. The mechanistic view presents human beings as divisible, predictable, and manageable, just like the machines and technologies that have become so prevalent in health care. Despite the many attempts to integrate caring practices and human values into this single image, mechanism prevails. Rather than being viewed separately, as beings with distinct and coexisting realities, persons have been conceptualized as consisting of parts and variables that must be observed, assessed, examined, managed, and controlled. These beliefs about human beings formed the foundation of modern science.

THE EMERGENCE OF OPPOSING PARADIGMS

From the earliest records of human thought there have been struggles and tensions between the opposing views depicting, on the one hand, knowledge of the natural world, and on the other, knowledge of human experiences, activities, and institutions. Isaiah Berlin (1997) offers a discerning overview of the struggles among persons who debated different ways of knowing in his book *Against the Current: Essays in the History of Ideas*. According to Berlin (1997), many thinkers through the ages have questioned ways of knowing, but Vico, in the 1700s, was the first philosopher to make explicit contrasts between the natural (mechanistic) and the human sciences. Berlin presents Vico's description of the schism that signaled a parting of ways over scientific views, and these contrasts continue to divide rather than unite the nursing community. Consider the following description of Vico's contrasts.

The specific and unique versus the repetitive and the universal, the concrete versus the abstract, perpetual movement versus rest, the inner versus the outer, quality versus quantity, culture-bound versus timeless principles, mental strife and self transformation as a permanent condition of man versus the possibility (and desirability) of peace, order, final harmony and the satisfaction of all rational human wishes. (Berlin, 1997, p. 109)

Vico's contributions to human science link with his insights into knowledge about human beings, knowledge that is possible because of the interrelationships among shared experience, imagination, and personal reality. Understanding what it is to hope, to fear, to believe in a cause, to have friends, to appreciate music, or to belong to a community is a kind of personal knowing that cannot be understood from some outside source, claimed Vico. Following Vico, there were other philosophers like Hamann, Kierkegaard, Herder, Jacobi, Schelling, and Bergson, to name several. These authors, from various angles, thrashed the rationalistic, objective, deterministic tenets of the natural sciences. Hamann referred to scientific systems as:

monstrous bureaucratic machines, built in accordance with the rules that ignore the teeming variety of the living world, the untidy and asymmetrical inner lives of men, and crush them into conformity for the sake of some ideological chimera unrelated to the union of spirit and flesh that constitutes the real world. (Berlin, 1997, p. 8)

Similarly, Herder described the existence of multiple, incommensurable cultures, and he wrote about the "false mechanical model" of mankind (Berlin, 1997, p. 12). Two hundred years after Vico first compared the natural and human sciences, Dilthey (1961, 1976, 1977, 1988), called for a human science that would honor lived experience and that would counter the sterility and lifeless void of the natural sciences.

More than calling for attention to human science, Dilthey addressed the complexity of coexisting realities, coexisting sciences, that as described may be consistent with the phenomenon of the pictures of paradox offered here. For instance, Dilthey wrote of a life-nexus, which was the place where the human being and the natural world connect while remaining separate in one person. He was interested in explicating how two philosophical and opposing paradigms relate with each other. Dilthey proposed that the subjective-objective dichotomy was non-existent in his notion of lived experience. For Dilthey (1961, 1976, 1977, 1988), human beings were seen as existing in a natural world understood through the senses, but he also claimed that human beings themselves could not be reduced to or derived from the natural world. From Dilthey's perspective, natural science and human science, and human and world, retained their separateness, and they also possessed a reciprocal interplay, a correlative togetherness; it is this togetherness, this life-nexus of paradigms that he focused on. Whatever people experience in the natural world can only be known through lived experience, proposed Dilthey. Further, for Dilthey, natural science described cause–effect relations among objects but only human science could situate those relations in the larger context of meanings, values, and purposes.

The importance of touching on the history of the ongoing struggle between the human science and the natural science or mechanistic paradigms is to enhance understanding of how we have arrived at this place in nursing where two scientific paradigms are seen as either incompatible or as one merged reality. It is understandable that nurses developed practice and research methodologies that contributed to the belief that there is only one credible view of reality. Many nursing students, for instance, have not been given the opportunity to engage the debates and the struggles about what can and cannot be understood when different views of reality coexist. Nurses have not had opportunities to move beyond the single view of reality, to see the picture of paradox, the coexisting paradigms about human beings, that are there awaiting discovery. This is so because most nurses, like other students, have been indoctrinated, especially over the past 50 years, with one view of reality, one preferred way of knowing, and that knowing is consistent with the mechanistic paradigm (Grudin, 1996; Hiraki, 1992; McIntyre, 1995). Grudin (1996) described the monistic, mechanistic tone in Western discourse that gets "passed on to the young as the proper way of thinking" (p. 15). Nurses, too, have been instructed in the so-called "proper way" that Grudin calls mechanistic logic. Mechanistic logic looks for simplistic answers to complex questions and it limits and obstructs thinking that embraces or represents the reality of complex lived experience.

A review of current textbooks commonly used in undergraduate nursing education reveals the almost total absence of content related to the substantive struggle and contributions of the mechanistic and human science paradigms. Typically, undergraduate nursing texts focus on physiology, pathophysiology, assessment, and intervention. For example, a 1,500-page text on medical-surgical nursing by Black and Matassarin-Jacobs (1997) offers no discussion of human science or scientific paradigms. Consistent with the mechanistic model, the text focuses on problems and interventions aimed at fixing problems. The authors rely on non-nursing theories to describe human beings. Interestingly, there is one description of the idea that nurses should respect others' freedom and be non-judgmental. Under the area of spiritual care, the authors suggest, "Accepting others as they are—without the traditional concern for defining, controlling, and changing—permits the spirit to expand and express itself" (Black & Matassarin-Jacobs, 1997, p. 73). Black and Matassarin-Jacobs do not, however, discuss the obvious paradox of guiding nurses to judge and control people, on the one hand, while accepting others so that the spirit can expand, on the other. Consistent with the reductionistic focus on human bio-psycho-social-sexual parts, the text offers literally hundreds of assessments and interventions. Some of the recommended assessments are particularly striking. For instance, the authors recommend that nurses ask people, "Have you ever wished you were of the opposite sex?" (p. 192). The arrogance and disrespect for the person in this question is hopefully obvious to the reader, and it demonstrates the extent to which nurses are taught to disregard human beings and their personal realities.

Two other nursing texts do present some content that suggests knowledge is underpinned by more than one science. Potter and Perry (1997), in their 1,500-page text on the fundamentals of nursing, included a very cursory discussion of nursing models, but the majority of the text supports a mechanistic approach, meaning they primarily describe nursing as the diagnosis and treatment of human responses to health. The authors refer to a melding of knowledge but there is no mention of paradigms or human science. Similarly, Clark (1996), in her text *Nursing in the Community*, describes several nursing theories. However, they are presented in the final chapter and are prefaced with the following caveat: "The epidemiolgic prevention process model around which this book is organized may not meet the needs of every community health nurse in every situation. For that reason, this final unit discusses several other models that may be useful" (Clark, 1996, p. 877). In Clark's thinking, the options for thinking and knowing about community health are presented in an either-or framework, as opposed to the notion of coexisting paradigms that inform and direct.

Obviously, the basic texts in nursing education do not do service to the important debate between the mechanistic and human science paradigms. Most nurses are subject to the monistic, mechanistic logic referred to above by Grudin (1996). The proposed reasons for the lack of attention to the well-developed debates about paradigms and practices restrict nurses and their right to struggle with the issues and to discover the opportunities that can flow from different ways of thinking about and being with patients. I have heard educators and other nursing leaders say that undergraduate nurses should not be confused with options. The consequence of this belief denies nurses the opportunity to become reflective and to expand ways of being with people; ways that honor lived experience and human freedom.

The absence of opportunity to engage the debate and wrestle with the opposing views of different paradigms has, in nursing, been restrictive in the extreme. The restriction shows itself in the ways nurses have extended the ideas of the mechanistic paradigm to the whole human being and his or her life. Specifically, beliefs about technology have extended into nursing's way of being with human beings and it is this way of being, this technologic stance, that is threatening and limiting nurses' opportunities to evolve and knowingly contribute to human quality of life. The harm of technology and the mechanistic model is told in stories and accounts from patients who engage health care professionals and who experience the judgmental disregard inherent with practices guided by the mechanistic paradigm. Deegan (1993), for example, wrote her moving account of what it was like to be labeled as a schizophrenic and treated in ways that left her feeling trapped in a web of surveillance and judgment. Another patient offered his views of what was not helpful during an acute mental illness. He stated that the following things were not helpful to him as a patient:

When therapists and institutions relied too heavily on medications, assuming that basic maintenance and waiting for the biochemical magic to take effect was enough. When nobody took the time to share my world with me and bring me into theirs. When the closest thing to human interaction was the drone of a television set, constantly turned to one station while the staff invisibly performed their institutional duties. When hospitals, modeled after prisons in so many respects, focused more on their own efficiency than on their healing missions . . . where nurses have time only to push their carts down the hall, dispensing "meds" like stewardesses passing out whisky and peanuts to passengers. (Edwards, 1997, p. 50)

The mechanistic paradigm and its related culture of technology have been evolving for several hundred years, and their influence in nursing, like other health-related disciplines, is far-reaching; so much so that the explicit and implicit assumptions and beliefs about human beings are no longer even recognized. The mechanistic beliefs have become culture and are embedded in the customs, habits, words, and thoughts of nurses. Recent efforts by some nurse leaders to reduce nursing practice to that which is evidence-based is symbolic of the pervasive influence of mechanistic beliefs in nursing. Evidence-based practice diminishes freedom and dignity for both nurses and clients. Honoring the freedom to think, to struggle with conflicting values, and to make choices based on personal knowledge, hopes, and desires are the things that define human life and professional nursing. Authors advocating for evidence-based practice as the initiative that will bring nurses greater control and management of people reinforce the myopic focus and disregard inherent in the mechanistic paradigm.

THE MECHANISTIC DISREGARD OF HUMANS

The central issue of concern surrounding technology and its related mechanistic framework is the disregard of human beings that directs nurses' thinking and acting with patients and families. As noted above, an essential feature of the mechanistic paradigm is that human beings are conceptualized in component parts or divisions. These divisions of humans were constructed, I believe, in order to facilitate the study and management of patients. The flaw in this reasoning is that although machines can be studied in parts and managed in function, human beings cannot. Nurses who believe they can manage people and their experiences of health have extended the knowledge of technology and endow human beings with machine-like qualities. This is true even when authors have attempted to integrate caring values and the words "human science."

For instance, Jones and Alexander (1993) developed the notion of "caring as technology" in an attempt to humanize the mechanistic view of technology. The authors, who rely on background definitions of technology as actions taken with or without tools, define caring as a technology that "is performed from one to another . . . to bring about some change in the recipient of technology" (Jones & Alexander, 1993, p. 18). The authors go on to state, "If technology is the practical application of science, and if the focus of nursing, as a human science, is caring, then the technology of caring can also be thought of as the practical application of human science" (p. 18). Despite the admirable intentions of these authors to preserve the values of human science, they fail to accomplish a sustainable model for their synthesis. Although Jones and Alexander contend there is a way to synthesize caring and technology, it is apparent in their presentation that the intent of their technology of caring is to change the recipient of the interaction, a notion consistent only with the mechanistic model of nursing care.

My point in disclaiming the synthesis proposed by Jones and Alexander can be demonstrated by returning to the notion of the picture of paradox. If you recall, in the picture of paradox one image becomes a totally different image when persons shift their view, yet each image is preserved in its uniqueness and in the thinking of the viewer who knows that each paradigm is there in its entirety. Jones and Alexander continue to see one view, despite their claim to the contrary. It is as if they place a mask over the mechanistic image and claim it is a different view of reality. But on close examination, their preferred view can be seen under the mask. It is there in their assumptions about human beings. Jones and Alexander assume that people can be changed and they assume the nurse's intent is to do the changing. These views are inconsistent with human science beliefs, which propose that the nurse's intent is to honor the changing of others without trying to determine the meaning or direction of the change (Parse, 1987, 1998).

A second essential feature of mechanistic science is comparison and judgment. Machines and procedures can be tested and refined so that function is optimized. When dealing with machines, there are standards of good that facilitate comparison in light of function, durability, efficiency, and so on. However, the notion that people too can be compared in light of function, durability, and efficiency is not only faulty, it is a harmful notion. Nurses who refer to people as unrealistic, abnormal, or dysfunctional are using biomedical language to represent what they see when they look at patients and families. Nursing diagnoses based on judgments of what is good or bad about human health are consistent with the mechanistic paradigm.

A third feature of mechanistic science and its disregard for humanity links to the issue of control. As noted above, the vast majority of nursing literature is directed at helping nurses believe they can manage human beings and their lived experiences of health, illness, living, and dying. For example, nurses who expect people to comply with goals that have not been defined by people themselves are working from within the mechanistic framework; or, predefined practice guidelines about what to teach based on a diagnosis are consistent only with the mechanistic paradigm. Approaches and practices like these dominate the nursing literature.

Nurses, like other health care practitioners, have been encouraged to blur the boundaries between physiology and life, between technology and humanity (Crawshaw, 1983). Human life has been turned into a cornucopia of physiological and behavioral variables that some nurses think can be isolated, measured, and controlled in the same ways technology can be monitored and controlled. Any call for nurses to be caring or empathic when viewing these variables fails to reveal the paradoxical paradigm of human science. Certainly, it is important for nurses to know how to follow procedures and protocols. But human beings, the living persons for whom nurses care, do not require such technologically inspired inspections and controls. Until nurses are able to knowingly shift their view between the mechanistic paradigm and the human science paradigm, they will not be able to advance or perform nursing as a human science and art as well as a practice discipline in the world of technology.

Given the inadequacies of the mechanistic model, one is left questioning what might help nurses to see the coexisting views of different realities. Nurses have primarily relied on authors from other disciplines to try to bring human experience and human values into the mechanistic picture. Buber, Frankl, Rogers, and Maslow have all received extensive coverage in nursing's educational programs. But it is as if the theories and values that nurses borrowed from other disciplines were simply considered from within the primary image of nursing as a mechanistic science. To return to the picture of paradox, most nurses who call for holistic practice or the integration of caring in nursing do so by adding details to the dominant image of mechanism, as opposed to creating a paradoxical and distinct image of nursing as a human science. The majority of nurses do not yet embrace the notion that nursing is a basic science. Nurses require nursing theories to coexist with other scientific beliefs and to create the insights of paradoxical shifts in thinking. Although nurses have addressed the inherent dangers of technology and its harmful extensions into the nurse–person relationship (see, for example, Pillar, Jacox, & Redman, 1990; Sandelowski, 1993, 1997, 1998), they have not yet dedicated sufficient attention to developing nursing theories consistent with the human science paradigm.

EMBRACING A PICTURE OF PARADOX FOR NURSING SCIENCE

A human science knowledge base that holds as much depth and clarity as the contrasting culture of technology is essential for nursing practice and research. The theory most familiar to this current author is Parse's (1981, 1998) theory of human becoming. Nurses who integrate the principles of human becoming learn how to practice in the presence of multiple views of reality—simultaneously. From Parse's view, the primary context of nursing is the nurse–person process where the priority of being truly present with others, as they live their health and becoming, complements the technologic requirements of modern-day nursing. First and foremost, nurses are called to fulfill their mandate to enhance quality of living through meaningful partnerships with others. Technological knowledge also guides nurses in their everyday practice, but the nurse is able to shift the view of reality in order to preserve the coexisting view of unitary human beings who continuously choose and change. In many settings, like hospitals, nurses participate in the delivery of technologic/physiologic care and in these situations they rely on the most up-to-date knowledge in order to promote clinical excellence. Technical competence, however, does not make a nurse. Many nurses are technically competent and valued as such, but so are other professionals. Even family members and patients/clients themselves are, or can become, technically skilled.

Technological knowledge is fleeting and ever changing; it is not owned by any group and informs many in modern health care. Technology will continue to revolutionize health care and self-care. Indeed, technology will free clients from dependence on professionals who have in the past controlled technical knowledge and its applications. Technology and evidence inform multiple groups in the context of certain physiological challenges, but this kind of knowledge cannot inform the nurse–person process, which must be guided by human science. Nurses are encouraged to find ways to create, and hold in view, the multiple paradigms of science that define the discipline. Mechanistic practices that do not coexist with human science threaten the nurse–person process and diminish opportunities for meaningful practices that focus on enhancing quality of life from the perspectives of persons themselves. If nursing is a unique art and science it must have a view of reality consistent with nursing's mandate to be helpful and life-enhancing.

The art and science of nursing are about knowing when to shift and how to preserve the coexisting paradigms that inform practice and research. In 1986, Barger-Lux and Heaney proposed that nurses might be the ones in systems to represent the patients' interests and provide a voice of compassion and common sense in light of the technological imperative that blinds many physicians. This opportunity does exist, and some nurses are choosing this path. The picture of paradox is a useful way to contemplate the unity and the distinctions among paradigms of science in nursing. There remains the possibility of other pictures of understanding yet hidden from view. Words to describe the ways paradigms coexist and direct thinking and acting are admittedly inadequate at this point. Clearly, some nurses are able to see and shift among multiple views of reality, and they do this in ways that show a seamless way of knowing and acting consistent with two paradigms of nursing science. Hopefully, nurses will continue to search for ways of understanding the complexities of paradox, paradigms, and nursing science.

REFERENCES

Baier, S. (1996). The view from bed number ten. *Healthcare Forum Journal, 39*, 60–67.

Barger-Lux, M. J., & Heaney, R. P. (1986). For better and worse: The technological imperative in health care. *Social Science & Medicine, 12*, 1313–1320.

Berlin, I. (1997). *Against the current: Essays in the history of ideas* (H. Hardy, Ed.). London: Pimlico.

Bernardo, A. (1998). Technology and true presence in nursing. *Holistic Nursing Practice, 12*(4), 40–49.

Black, J. M., & Matassarin-Jacobs, E. (1997). *Medical-surgical nursing: Clinical management for continuity of care* (5th ed.). Philadelphia: W. B. Saunders.

Clark, M. J. (1996). *Nursing in the community* (2nd ed.). Stamford, CT: Appleton & Lange.

Crawshaw, R. (1983). Technical zeal or therapeutic purpose—How to decide? *Journal of the American Medical Association, 250*, 1857–1859.

Deegan, P. (1993). Recovering our sense of value after being labeled. *Journal of Psychosocial Nursing, 31*(4), 4–11.

Deveaux, B., & Babin, S. (1994). [Review of the Canadian Broadcasting Corporation documentary *Not My Home*]. Deveaux-Babin Productions.

Deveaux, B., & Babin, S. (1996). [Review of the production *Real Stories*]. Deveaux-Babin Productions.

Dilthey, W. (1961). *Pattern and meaning in history: Thoughts on history and society* (H. P. Rickman, Trans.). New York: Harper and Row.

Dilthey, W. (1976). *Selected writings* (H. P. Rickman, Trans.). Cambridge: Cambridge University Press.

Dilthey, W. (1977). *The understanding of other persons and their expressions of life* (Original work published 1927). In R. M. Zaner & K. L. Heiges (Trans.),

Descriptive psychology and historical understanding (pp. 123–144). The Hague, Netherlands: Nijhoff.

Dilthey, W. (1988). *Introduction to the human sciences* (R. J. Betanzos, Trans.). Detroit: Wayne State University Press. (Original work published 1883).

Edwards, C. (1997). Understand. In J. Young-Mason, (Ed.), *The patient's voice: Experience of Illness.* (pp. 49–53). Philadelphia: F. A. Davis.

Fisher, M. (1994). *Sleep with the angels.* London: Moyer Bell.

Gadow, S. (1984). Touch and technology: Two paradigms of patient care. *Journal of Religion and Health, 23,* 63–69.

Gerteis, M., Edgman-Levitan, S., Daley, J., & Delbanco, T. (Eds.). (1993). *Through the patient's eyes. Understanding and promoting patient-centered care.* San Francisco: Jossey-Bass.

Giorgi, A. (1970). *Psychology as a human science.* New York: Harper and Row.

Giorgi, A. (1985). Sketch of a psychological phenomenological method. In A. Giorgi (Ed.), *Phenomenology and psychological research* (pp. 8–22). Pittsburgh: Duquesne University Press.

Grudin, R. (1996). *On dialogue.* Boston: Houghton Mifflin.

Guba, E. G., & Lincoln, Y. S. (1990). Can there be a human science? *Person-Centered Review, 5,* 130–154.

Hiraki, A. (1992). Tradition, rationality, and power in introductory nursing textbooks: A critical hermeneutics study. *Advances in Nursing Science, 14*(3), 1–12.

Jones, C. B., & Alexander, J. W. (1993). The technology of caring: A synthesis of technology and caring for nursing administration. *Nursing Administration Quarterly, 17*(2), 11–20.

Kim, H. S. (2000). An integrative framework for conceptualizing clients: A proposal for a nursing perspective in the new century. *Nursing Science Quarterly, 13,* 37–40.

Locsin, R. C. (1995). Machine technologies and caring in nursing. *Image: Journal of Nursing Scholarship, 27,* 201–203.

Macurdy, A. H. (1997). Mastery of life. In J. Young-Mason, (Ed.), *The patient's voice: Experience of Illness.* (pp. 9–17). Philadelphia: F. A. Davis.

McConnell, E. A. (1998). The coalescence of technology and humanism in nursing practice: It doesn't just happen and it doesn't come easily. *Holistic Nursing Practice, 12*(4), 23–30.

McIntyre, M. (1995). "The focus of the discipline of nursing": A critique and extension. *Advances in Nursing Science, 18*(1), 27–35.

Mitchell, G. J., & Cody, W. K. (1992). Nursing knowledge and human science: Ontological and epistemological considerations. *Nursing Science Quarterly, 5,* 54–61.

Mitchell, G. J., & Lawton, C. (2000). Living with the consequences of personal choices for persons with diabetes: Implications for educators and practitioners. *Canadian Journal of Diabetes Care, 24*(2), 23–31.

Nagle, L. M. (1998). The meaning of technology for people with chronic renal failure. *Holistic Nursing Practice, 12*(4), 78–92.

Newman, M. (1994). *Health as expanding consciousness* (2nd ed.). New York: National League for Nursing Press.

Parse, R. R. (1981). *Man-living-health: A theory of nursing.* New York: Wiley.

Parse, R. R. (1987). *Nursing science: Major paradigms, theories and critiques*. Philadelphia: Saunders.

Parse, R. R. (1998). *The human becoming school of thought: A perspective for nurses and other health professionals*. Thousand Oaks, CA: Sage.

Parse, R. R. (1999). Nursing science: The transformation of practice. *Journal of Advanced Nursing, 30*, 1383–1387.

Pillar, B., Jacox, A. K., & Redman, B. K. (1990). Technology, its assessment, and nursing. *Nursing Outlook, 38*, 16–19.

Polkinghorne, D. E. (1988). *Narrative knowing and the human sciences*. Albany: State University of New York Press.

Potter, P. A., & Perry, A. G. (1997). *Canadian fundamentals of nursing* (J. R. Kerr & M. K. Sirotnik, Eds.). St. Louis, MO: Mosby.

Rawnsley, M. M. (2000). Response to Kim's human living concept as a unifying perspective for nursing. *Nursing Science Quarterly, 13*, 41–44.

Ray, M. A. (1987). Technological caring: A new model in critical care. *Dimensions in Critical Care Nursing, 6*, 166–173.

Sandelowski, M. (1993). Toward a theory of technology dependency. *Nursing Outlook, 41*, 36–42.

Sandelowski, M. (1997). (Ir)Reconcilable differences? The debate concerning nursing and technology. *Image: Journal of Nursing Scholarship, 29*, 169–174.

Sandelowski, M. (1998). Looking to care or caring to look? Technology and the rise of spectacular nursing. *Holistic Nursing Practice, 14*(4), 1–11.

Schroeder, C. (1998). So this is what it's like: Struggling to survive in pediatric intensive care. *Advances in Nursing Science, 20*(4), 13–22.

Szawarski, Z. (1989). Dignity and technology. *The Journal of Medicine and Philosophy, 14*, 243–249.

Watson, J. (1985). *Nursing: Human science and human care*. Norwalk, CT: Appleton-Century-Crofts.

Watson, J. (1995). Nursing's caring-healing paradigm as exemplar for alternative medicine. *Alternative Therapies, 1*(3), 64–69.

Young-Mason, J. (1997). *The patient's voice: Experiences of illness*. Philadelphia: F. A. Davis.

Chapter 4

Complex Culture and Technology: Toward a Global Caring Communitarian Ethics of Nursing

Marilyn A. Ray

INTRODUCTION

New forms of ethical understanding are necessary in an increasingly complex, technologic, and culturally dynamic universe. Today we are in a cultural reformation called globalization, initiated in part by the communication age and fueled by advanced technology and economic progress or greed (Mander & Goldsmith, 1996). The technologies of the Internet, cellular phones, cable television, and airline transportation have made the world and people closer. Where technology dominates through the computer, fax, and the Internet, as in world governments, particularly Western, in academia, and in businesses, "electro-personal/corporate" values have been introduced. The Internet has created the situation for a network of people to communicate with each other without meeting or seeing each other face-to-face. This technological community is creating new ethical challenges for communities. The information or communication age has brought people of diverse cultures closer together but, paradoxically, at the same time has driven them apart. Fear of control by Western cultures and concern for the loss of cultural identities with traditional ideologies, specific religious values, and unique ways of life is growing. Moreover, health care systems all over the world are caught in the throes of the economics of care whereby populations desperately try to get basic primary care but also try to reap the advantages of technological care, including advanced pharmacotherapeutics. The potential negative and positive effects of the power of the advancing economic and technological globalization continue to pose as challenges for nurses internationally. The processes of globalization often impact people negatively in terms of health, brought about by reorganization of communities, changes in cultural belief systems, poverty of body, mind, and spirit, and devastation of the environment. Without knowledge and opportunities for participating in the ethical debate at local and global levels regarding health care politics and policy development, nurses will have only the remnants of others' decisions with which to engage. Nurses who are most capable of advocacy on the nurse–client level can also act on the communal level. A global nursing ethics grounded in caring and communitarianism is necessary to awaken nurses to the ethical responsibilities as cultures fuse or converge. This chapter focuses on an approach to understanding globalization in culture and health care, and introduces a complexity of transcultural caring and a communitarian ethics as frameworks for application in culturally dynamic caring situations.

TECHNOLOGY, CULTURE, AND HUMAN VALUES

Barbour (1980) reported that the 1960s began with high confidence in technology in the United States and other Western nations. The evolution of the space age, computer and health care technologies, and the quest for economic or material well-being were achievements of technological ingenuity. In the United States, technological progress, the triumph over nature, and material consumption were the dream, resulting in personal fulfillment or seeking the "good life." By the end of the 1960s, however, there was growing concern about the social and environmental impacts of technology, namely, social isolation and damage to the natural environment. In developing countries, crises were even more profound. Economic and technological growth had benefited privileged minorities and the basic needs of vast majorities were not met. Environmental and human costs ensued despite improvements in health care, agricultural productivity, and efforts to abate pollution of the air, soil, and water (Mander & Goldsmith, 1996; Mesthane, 1983b).

History has shown that cultures are radically altered by the revolutionary changes in science and technology. A technological universe exemplifies this change. Mesthene (1983a, 1983b) claimed that new technology means enhancing our ability to measure, predict, control, or direct *and* simultaneously create new possibilities as a result of uncertainty and unpredictability. Technology therefore alters our mix of choices. Older possibilities are displaced or prior choices are reversed by altering the spectrum of options and mix or hierarchy of social choices. Different cultures committed to different values react differently to the same new technological possibilities. The central characteristics of dynamic culture are change and renewal. By constantly renewing themselves, cultures can preserve unique identities while balancing the coalescing of human beings with complex social and technological environments. Subsequently, the question is, "What should we do and particularly what should we do when we are a 'company of strangers' sharing a common world?" (Palmer, 1981). How should culture and technology be defined? Swerdlow (1999) endorsed the remarks of the geographer, Peter Jackson, that cultures are maps of meaning through which the world is made intelligible (pp. 4–5). Culture is the foundation from which people in relationship can find the means necessary for its growth and development. Culture, thus, is dynamic, complex, and relational. People of diverse cultures form the foundation for participation in creating and responding to the meaning of relationships—human, spiritual, social, and material. Conflicting values and priorities provide opportunities for thoughtful reflection and choices as cultures converge and attempt to form a coherent community with which to build the global civic culture (Boulding, 1988). "The commitment to universal intelligibility [global community] entails moral responsibility" (Mesthene, 1983a, p. 115).

THE PHILOSOPHICAL BASIS OF COMMUNITY

Before we can move toward a development or restoration of a moral voice of community, and nursing's voice and activity in it, there is a need to examine the meaning of community. Community has many definitions. Kirkpatrick (1986) identified over 90 views ranging from nature, quest, search, and the theological basis of community to community as location of a cultural meaning system. Culture transmits the values and attitudes that hinder or create community.

Kirkpatrick (1986) identified three philosophical models of community: atomistic-contractarian, organic-functional, and mutual-personal. In addition, the information and genetic ages have given us new models—the virtual community (Rheingold, 1993) and the biotechnical community (Rifkin, 1996) which now dominate our global politics, economics, health care, and agricultural arenas.

Atomistic-Contractarian Model of Community

Atomistic-contractarian philosophy postulates that forms of human association are based on contracts, and that society is composed of independent atoms or individual entities who rationally contract with each other for the terms of their enforced relationship. The metaphysical assumption is that free individuals in a state of unimpeded self-interest enter into a contractual arrangement for self-protection (Kirkpatrick, 1986). Priority is given to the individual rather than to the group because the state of nature is such that no real group exists. The function of the state is to secure good and provide defense against all others for the sake of the individual. Hobbes, Locke, Rousseau, Bentham, Mill, and Smith were the primary philosophers of atomistic-contractarianism. Their ideas were rooted in part in the traditions of Plato and Aristotle. From this philosophical view, they argued that social relationships were not only for self-protection but also for developing a person's higher faculties toward the enhancement of others. The commitment to individualism has played a major role in Britain, Europe, and North America, but has had the most decisive influence on American culture (Kirkpatrick, 1986).

Organic-Functional Model of Community

A group of interdependent, functionally related organs within a larger organism is the metaphor of the organic-functional model of community. This model arose in response to the deficiencies identified as isolationist within the atomistic-contractarian model. The metaphysical assumption within this view is Marxian, which posits that persons create a human community by activating their fundamental nature, that is, they are social beings (Kirkpatrick, 1986). Moreover, from a philosophical perspective advocated by Hegel and Whitehead, relationality, pieces, and differentiated parts must not impair the unity or totality of the organism as a whole. From a Hegelian viewpoint, the unity of the whole emphasized the interrelatedness of reality. In this model, the center of social philosophy shifted from the individual to the community. Marxian advocacy established socialistic, political, and economic associations as alternatives to capitalistic ideology by appealing to interdependence and cooperation among individuals. These understandings of community were to the atomistic perspective, the germ of totalitarianism, or the notion that "the individual is the pawn of the state" (Kirkpatrick, 1986, p. 69). Although Marxist theory showed the importance of the interrelationship of persons, nature, ideas, and social and economic structures, the attempt to remove the barriers to self-determination and the egoism of atomistic thought prevented an exploration of how persons-in-relation freely choose their ends or goals, specifically relationships of love and mutuality (Kirkpatrick, 1986).

Mutual-Personal Model of Community

While the atomistic-contractarian and the organic-functional models of community present a central problem desirous of reconciling the issue of individual goals of freedom and self-interest, and for the reconciliation of interpersonal and social relationships, Kirkpatrick (1986) declared the mutual-personal model of community as the ultimate avenue. Such a model depicts a vision of mutuality in which individuals find fulfillment in and through living for each other in loving fellowship. The person is not sacrificed at the expense of the community. The process of entering into community is a personal moral choice—what one person does, either by way of help or hindrance, affects the actions of others. The communal mode of relationship, a unity of persons as persons, maintained by mutual affection, love, or friendship, is the only positively motivated form of relation.

The Virtual and Biotechnical/Biocolonization Communities

The computer and Internet have created the opportunity for a network of people to communicate with each other without meeting or seeing each other face-to-face, the faceless or virtual community. People log on to the computer and Internet at any time to give or receive information on any subject with a company of strangers who could be referred to as "info-face" friends with "electro-personal/corporate" values.

Moreover, the biotechnical or biocolonization community has created an intriguing approach to reality. On the positive side, biotechnology is a rapidly growing field, producing new treatments for a variety of diseases ranging from diabetes mellitus to various cancers. Biotechnology integrates microbiology, immunology, genetics, molecular biology, and biochemistry for diagnosing, treating, and preventing disease (Schrand, 1999). On the negative side, many scientists, economists, or corporations are in competition with each other and attempting to lay claim to the genetic foundation of nature that Kimbrell (1996) calls the marketeers of life. Genetic engineering and reengineering through advanced technologies and economic control are creating a variety of transgenic animals and plants, a global market in body parts, and what could be called the end of nature (Kimbrell, 1996). Boulding (1988) discussed the building of a global civic culture in the "company of strangers" (Palmer, 1981)—those who share a common space, common resources, and common opportunities. The virtual community fulfills this definition through cyberspace technological networks of information.

Deep conflicts and ethical questions, however, have arisen in the biotechnical community, between nature and nurture, between the alteration in foundations of life for economic gain and the nurturing of human persons with moral reasoning for the good of society (Rifkin, 2000). Unique problems in terms of the moral realm emerge with questions like the following: Are there common ethical values that hold an information and biotechnical society together? What is the quality of humanness or friendships developed through machines or relationships? How does one know the meaning of authenticity or truth through faceless or info-face technology? How are aging, health, and health care changing with biotechnology? Can there be such a thing as a biodemocracy?

THE EVOLVING MEANING OF COMMUNITY

According to Cohen (1985/1989), community is a cultural meaning system and is seen as arising in consciousness, or the mind and experience (past, present, and future potential). Community as a bearer of meaning can be used as a model of reality to interpret the familiar and unfamiliar (Geertz, 1973). Thus, symbolically constructed and boundaryless, community as a cultural meaning system provides a sense of identity and belongingness for its members. This boundaryless view, oriented to consciousness, challenges ideas which emphasized community as highly structured either in socioeconomic class, ethnicity, racial group, or as nations with specific ideologies. Recognized as a symbolic whole of interconnected and multicultural human relationships, boundaryless meaning systems transcend individualistic cultural forces. Strict political ideologies of socialism and capitalism become blurred and less relevant. Moreover, in the wake of global political, economic, and technological interdependence, reliance on the goodwill, caring, and moral commitment of national leaders and professional practitioners becomes greater. Today, the living of community must be constituted not only by emphasis on individual or particular group rights, but by a new meaning of community with commitment to belongingness, mutuality, and communitarianism (Christians, Ferre, & Fackler, 1994; White, 1996), emphasizing moral voices that speak for the good of others.

AN EMERGING NURSING ETHICS: GLOBAL CARING COMMUNITARIAN ETHICS

Where does nursing fit into these visions of community? How will nursing address the issues that are emerging in globalization and global corporate culture? How will nursing deal with the dynamic global culture evolving through technology? How will nursing understand the meaning of human values in the postmodern age? How will nursing cocreate a new global ethical vision of reality to participate in building a global civic culture and the culture of peace? (Boulding, 1988). Professional nursing ethics has always focused attention on the good—doing good for the society through providing nursing care. Professional codes of ethics, such as the American Nurses Association (ANA) Code for Nurses or the International Council of Nurses Code for Nurses (1973) make explicit the goals and values of the profession (Benjamin & Curtis, 1992).

Deontology is one of the philosophical positions in professional ethics. Deontology deals with duties and obligations and articulates a set of norms which the professional must observe. Professionals must act not only in accordance with, but for the sake of the obligation to do good

(Alonso, 1996; Beauchamp & Childress, 1994). Utilitarianism or consequence-based theory has also been advanced in biomedical and nursing ethics. This position holds that actions are right or wrong according to the balance of their good and bad consequences, or the principle that we must always produce the maximal balance of positive value over the least possible disvalue (Beauchamp & Childress, 1994). Often there is a clash between the values associated with consequence and obligation; for example, nurses may act out of fear of consequences related to providing patient care rather than out of the sheer obligation to provide care.

The metaphor of culture as a "dynamic complexity" (Ray & Turkel, in process) in a world changed by the growth of technology and economics has value for an ethics of nursing (Davidson & Ray, 1991; Ray, 1994b, 1998b). Nursing, more than any other discipline, is involved with the dynamics of cultural complexity and the practice of relatedness through sociocultural interaction and the social structures co-created by people in cultures. The central concepts of complexity are interconnectedness, relationship, pattern recognition, and choice, as well as the paradoxes of determinism and non-determinism, predictability and non-predictability, causality and non-linearity, and disorder and order (Briggs & Peat, 1999; Wheatley, 1999). Nurses deal with all or aspects of these phenomena in caring for culturally diverse clients, families, and communities in practice.

While nursing culture may have changed over time, often as a result of inadequate answers to moral questions in practice (principally due to economic apprehension in corporate health care and technological overuse), caring and advocacy remain the foci of nursing worldwide (Gadow, 1988; Ray, 1994a, 1994b). As such, nurses are seeking to understand the meaning of networks of relationships by questioning immoral practice and reconnecting to others through caring. In clinical decision making, nurses have based their decisions on considerations of universal moral principles of doing good, and doing no harm, autonomy, justice, as well as advocacy. As knowledge changes through multicultural understanding, a global caring ethics is necessary. The emerging global caring communitarian ethic is grounded in the tenets of complexity science, transcultural caring, and communitarian ethics, which has the potential to lead to genuine cooperation, sharing, and choice-making around *common* values and *common* moral premises rather than the phenomena that divide (Ray, 1994a, 1994b; White, 1996). Both personal and communitarian decision making recognizes that diverse cultures must gain cultural capital—the recognition and affirmation that people of diverse identities can contribute to the development of a civil society (White, 1996).

Cultural capital thus involves the interplay among transcultural caring practices, ethical principles, the microsocial and macrosocial structural characteristics of diverse cultures (economic, technological, legal, political), and the universal sources or tenets of diverse religions that shape and are shaped by the exchange of cultural beliefs and experiences (Ray, 1994b). Transcultural/global caring includes acts of compassion and justice within a cultural context (Ray, 1989, 1994a). The most fundamental principle is respect for persons. Other principles include autonomy (self-determination), beneficence (doing good), non-maleficence (avoiding harm), veracity (truth-telling), confidentiality (respecting privileged information), fidelity (keeping promises), and justice (treating people fairly and fidelity to relationships) (ANA, 1985; Gadow, 1988; Ray, 1989, 1994b).

On the scientific-practical levels, complexity science, information technology, transcultural caring, and communitarianism can be the symbols through which nurses can co-create a global nursing ethics in the world for greater integration and wholeness of humanity. Nurses have the moral imperative, through diverse media, to use cultural capital to facilitate communal choice-making to reshape the vision of nursing, to maintain or establish coherence and a culture of peace in a changing world (Boulding, 1988). Ultimately, coherence rests with individual awareness of one's own experiences and knowledge of the world and one's place in it (Koerner, 1997). Increased knowledge of a personal, moral consciousness within a mutual, global consciousness is necessary.

THE PRACTICE OF GLOBAL CARING COMMUNITARIAN ETHICS

Globalization, multiculturalism, communication technology, and the biotechnical revolution are rapidly changing the way ethics in nursing and health care is practiced. New forms of ethics and health care/nursing ethics need to be considered. Given the transformation in world cultures, and the complexity of nursing science and art, traditional, principle-based nursing ethics must expand to include ideas advanced in complexity science and computer technology. Knowledge from the science of "change" unites seemingly contradictory constituents—interconnectedness and self-organization, non-linearity and determinism, and chaos (order and disorder). Co-creativeness through moral choice-making is the means to appreciate the value of co-evolution and cooperation, and is the holographic perspective of recognizing that the individual is part of the whole world culture and the whole world culture is in the individual. All individuals thus are part of each other—the mutual-personal community. We are transformed by communicative action (Habermas, 1987) and moral choice. Research and understanding of communicative action created by the technology revolution also are essential. Both individually and collectively, we advance through communication that is participatory, dialogical, horizontal, creative, and ethical (White, 1996). Communication that is relational is communitarian and facilitates moral choices brought about by having compassion for and understanding of unique cultural identities (racial, ethnic, religious, gender) (Davidson & Ray, 1991; Ray, 1994a, 1998b; Wheatley, 1999).

At the same time, communication that is conveyed technologically challenges us to deeper contemplation about the nature and meaning of relationships in complex society. A global caring communitarian ethics is a way to facilitate deeper contemplation. It acknowledges the realities occurring in a global culture. It affirms diverse cultural identities and encourages a participatory ethos and intense quest for understanding ethical public life, including the public life co-created through technological communication methods.

Communitarianism responds to a call to build a global civic culture in the company of strangers. Boulding (1988) remarked that the very concept of civic culture was borne out of experiences of conflict and diversity and comes from the Latin *civitas*, or city. Boulding stated that, historically, in cities, strangers came together at the convenience of kings. This company of strangers had to learn to communicate across language barriers and customs. They had to develop a set of understandings on how to exist and co-create in life to accomplish the act of living. Boulding stated that we must now examine all the diverse identities, to develop a shared civility across differences on a global scale in various civilizations and contemplate what the identity would look like.

The goal of a global caring communitarian ethics is not only making sure the voices of minorities are heard in public debate, but making sure that the subcultures gain cultural capital through the very technology (the Internet) that, because of their lack of knowledge, may even hold them back (White, 1996). Cultural capital focuses on the idea that immigrants or minorities are necessary for the revitalization and growth of a region or nation, rather than a liability, and that all groups can exist together to rebuild societies. In health care, for example, organization of people's health circles locally could represent the rights of the ill in relation to the structure of public and/or private health services.

The need exists to open a space in the public media (technology) for networks of organizations who defend the lifeworld of humanity. Opening the space requires the compassion of the public communicator, who can be not only a journalist or politician, but also a nurse. Nursing has the tradition of advocacy. By awareness and communicative action, nurses can help others to appreciate the experience of injustice, especially in the areas of health care access and social suffering. Nurses can communicate the sense of injustice to others. The starting point is entering into the complexity of articulating how the issues around cultural identities of different groups and health care can be confronted.

The nurse as communicator addressing a communitarian ethic must appeal to the values of society or societies and call for a reformulation of what the society presumes to be public cultural truth (White, 1995). What are the truth criteria for health or illness care, for example, in American society? The criteria for truthfulness using a global caring communitarian ethics should encompass the mutual-personal model of community, including a decided evaluation of what an ethical virtual community should be. It should acknowledge the ethics of compassion and justice, the common symbol of fidelity to and fairness in relationships, and fidelity to a sense of human dignity. It should acknowledge that even people who may not have access to technology to convey information can still be heard. A new form of global caring communitarianism needs dialogue to illuminate the great cultural traditions—racial and cultural identities, intricate historical processes, and institutionalization of good and bad habits that are a part of the social reality. The nurse as a public communicator or ethicist may run the risk of being ostracized by asking pointed questions that are the most delicate of all and reveal obvious but painful truths. However, to move toward a unity of intentions requires courage and moral choice.

When reflecting on the state of the world and the amount of evil that is perpetrated in the name of nations or relationships, it hardly seems that a model of compassion and justice could be central to the thinking of most people in institutions or governments. People agree that it is even difficult to live in loving fulfillment with their own families. At worst, we view one another as strangers where the other must be treated with distrust and fear because the other's self-interest may conflict with our own. At best, we see each other as friends, but only in spots; we are people of ambivalence (Viorst, 1986). But we can accept imperfect relationships. A global caring communitarianism is the knowledge and practice of relatedness. As nurses, we can promote a more ethical way of life that resonates with the wholeness of persons as world cultures change and grow. We can develop an ethical common sense.

CONCLUDING STATEMENTS

Nursing's distinctive position in the world in terms of the centrality of caring will facilitate a global caring communitarian ethics. The new ethics not only looks to individuals and their families to understand the meaning of cultural illness and health, but to the collective social, technological, political, and economic forces that encourage or discourage the development of well-being or wholeness. Virtual information and biotechnology within globalization challenge nurses to seek understanding of complex systems and how cultures can function together ethically in this age of rapid change. Global caring communitarianism responds to a relationship between compassion and justice in terms of what ought to be done within the dynamics of diverse cultures and technological societies (Ray, 1989). Compassion and justice as unique forms of human activity are the foundation of the moral character of community life itself. Global caring communitarian ethics is a way of nursing life that identifies patterns of relationships that facilitate cultural truth and moral choices, to promote health and healing and improve social conditions. As such, it is the heart of the mutual-personal community life. It is ethical common sense that will contribute to restoring the human factor to an ever-increasingly technological, and economically driven, world.

REFERENCES

Alonso, A. (1996). Seven theses on professional ethics. *Ethical Perspectives: Rethinking Professional Ethics, 3*(4), 200–206.

American Nurses Association (ANA). (1985). Code for nurses. Washington, DC: ANA.

Barbour, I. (1980). *Technology, environment, and human values.* New York: Praeger.

Beauchamp, T., & Childress, J. (1994). *Principles of biomedical ethics* (4th ed.). New York: Oxford University Press.

Benjamin, M., & Curtis, J. (1992). *Ethics in nursing* (3rd ed.). New York: Oxford University Press.

Boulding, C. (1988). *Building a global civic culture.* New York: Teachers College Press.

Briggs, J., & Peat, F. (1999). *Seven life lesson of chaos.* New York: HarperCollins Publishers.

Christians, C., Ferre, J., & Fackler, P. (1994). *Good news: Social ethics and the press.* New York: Oxford University Press.

Cohen, A. (1985/1989). *The symbolic construction of community.* New York: Routledge.

Davidson, A., & Ray, M. (1991). Studying the human-environment phenomenon using the science of complexity. *Advances in Nursing Science, 14*(2), 73–87.

Gadow, S. (1988). Covenant without cure: Letting go and holding on in chronic illness. In J. Watson & M. Ray (Eds.), *The ethics of care and the ethics of cure: Synthesis in chronicity* (pp. 5–14). New York: National League for Nursing.

Geertz, C. (1973). *The interpretation of culture.* New York: Basic Books.

Habermas, J. (1987). *The theory of communicative action,* Vol. 2 (T. McCarthy, Trans.). Boston: Beacon Press.

Kimbrell, A. (1996). Biocolonization: The patenting of life and the global market in body parts. In J. Mander & E. Goldsmith (Eds.), *The case against the global economy* (pp. 131–145). San Francisco: Sierra Club Books.

Kirkpatrick, F. (1986). *Community: A trinity of models.* Washington, DC: Georgetown University Press.

Koerner, J. (1997). Cocreation of culture through choice. In J. Dienemann (Ed.), *Cultural diversity in health care* (pp. 63–69). Washington, DC: American Academy of Nursing.

Locsin, R. (1995). Machine technologies. *Image: Journal of Nursing Scholarship, 27*(3), 201–203.

Mander, J., & Goldsmith, E. (Eds.). (1996). *The case against the global economy*. San Francisco: Sierra Club Books.

Mesthene, E. (1983a). How technology will shape the future. In C. Mitcham & R. Mackey (Eds.), *Philosophy and technology* (pp. 116–129). New York: The Free Press.

Mesthene, E. (1983b). Technology and wisdom. In C. Mitcham & R. Mackey (Eds.), *Philosophy and technology* (pp. 109–115). New York: The Free Press.

Palmer, P. (1981). *The company of strangers*. New York: Crossroad.

Ray, M. (1989). Transcultural caring: Political and economic visions. *Journal of Transcultural Nursing, 1*(1), 17–21.

Ray, M. (1994a). Communal moral experience as the research starting point for health care ethics. *Nursing Outlook, 42*(3), 104–109.

Ray, M. (1994b). Transcultural nursing ethics: A framework and model for transcultural ethical analysis. *Journal of Holistic Nursing, 12*(3), 251–264.

Ray, M. (1998a). The interface of caring and technology. A new reflexive ethics in intermediate care. *Holistic Nursing Practice, 12*(4), 69–77.

Ray, M. (1998b). Complexity and nursing science. *Nursing Science Quarterly, 11*(3), 91–93.

Ray, M., & Turkel, M. (in process). *Transcultural caring dynamics in nursing and health care*. Philadelphia: F. A. Davis Company.

Rheingold, H. (1993). *Virtual community*. Menlo Park, CA: Addison-Wesley.

Rifkin, J. (1996). New technology and the end of jobs. In J. Mander & E. Goldsmith (Eds.), *The case against the global economy* (pp. 108–121). San Francisco: Sierra Club Books.

Rifkin, J. (2000). *The biotechnology revolution*. Lecture, Florida Atlantic University, February 14.

Schrand, L. (1999). Recent additions to the growing biotechnological armamentarium: A critical assessment. *Formulary, 34*(11), 920–932.

Swerdlow, J. (Ed.). (1999). Global culture. *National Geographic, 196*(2), 2–11.

Viorst, J. (1986). *Necessary losses*. New York: Fawcett Gold Medal.

Wheatley, M. (1999). *Leadership and the new science* (2nd ed.). San Francisco: Berrett-Koehler.

White, R. (1995). From codes of ethics to public cultural truth: A systematic view of communication ethics. *European Journal of Communication, 10*(4), 441–459.

White, R. (1996). Communitarian ethic of communication in a postmodern age. *Ethical Perspectives: Rethinking Professional Ethics, 3*(4), 207–218.

Chapter 5

The Language of Nursing:
A Technology of Caring

Marguerite J. Purnell

But I can really show what I have in mind only by events which
open up into a genuine change from communication to communion,
that is, an embodiment of the word of dialogue. (Buber, 1965)

ONCE UPON A REPORT TIME

Inside the halls of evening, nurses of the day shift began the ritual of
"handing over" their patients to the oncoming night nurses. Pairs of
nurses sequestered themselves in quiet corners, each weary day nurse
giving rapid report and surrendering responsibility for patients to the
nurse just beginning the long evening shift.

One nurse began, "Patient is an 81-year-old male admitted to E.R.
complaining of tightness in chest, diaphoresis and nausea for three hours
before admittance. Denies chest pain. Blood pressure on admittance 85/
50, pulse irregular, ECG shows SVT." Continuing report in a time-
honored, rapid-fire routine, the nurse conveys patient data using "medicalese"—succinct, accurate medical terminology to convey chains of
information; patient medical history, medical interventions,
physiological status, and lab results. Nursing interventions and outcomes
were relayed in similar truncated fashion.

When the nurse had completed the medical description of the patient,
she leaned over, touching the other on the arm, and sought out eye
contact. "You know, I felt I really nursed today. He was so scared when
he came in—he thought he was going to die. He cried and I cried and
then talked him through it. We somehow connected. I got him laughing

afterwards—told him that nobody dares to die on my shift. He's old and alone, poor man—all his friends and family are dead. I guess he figures it's his turn now. He's OK, but keep an eye on him."

"My other patient is very different. He's a frequent flyer. Watch this one carefully. I know he's going to code, I just know it. His labs are within normal limits, everything seems OK, but there's something going on. I can't put my finger on it. . . . Let me give you report first." And the biomedical description began.

THE LANGUAGE OF NURSING: WHAT IS IT?

When nurses gather together for report, the frenetic and almost desperate event of change of shift takes place. The lives of those who are in their care become compressed into the impersonal phraseology of medicalese—the objective, quantitative, and calculable aspects of the patient's being that nurses must communicate to the next shift. Statistics, monitor strips, lab reports, fluids in, fluids out, measurements in grams, ounces, millimeters, and drops are translated by the nurse into an objective description of the patient's physical health. In the manner of medical case histories, biological processes are separated from the patients who experience them, and fundamental beliefs and values of the medical world are enacted (Anspach, 1994).

However, a distinct change in tenor occurs in the giving and receiving of report. The bimodal nature of nursing report becomes evident when nurses switch to communicating the reality of their nursing caring knowledge, their knowing, and their subjective experience. Medical terms and statistics, the objective shorthand of the health care industry, are conspicuously absent. Instead, nurses abruptly and naturally change to a vivid, human vernacular and present a description of the whole person. The patient is revealed as a suffering human being who is known by name, who cannot be divided into parts, and who thinks and feels and laughs and cries. Shift by shift, day by day, nurses communicate their caring practice. Yet what *is* the language of nursing?

Language is primarily defined as "a body of words and the systems for their use common to a people who are of the same community or nation, the same geographical area, or the same cultural tradition," and also as "the speech or phraseology peculiar to a class, profession, etc." (*Webster's Encyclopedic Unabridged Dictionary*, 1996, p. 1081). Speech is defined as "The faculty or power of speaking; oral communication; ability to express one's thoughts and emotions by speech sounds and gesture" (*Webster's*, 1996, p. 1833). While language is the set of conventions, speech, then, is more particularly the action of putting these conventions to use. Linguistics is "the science of language, including phonetics, phonology, morphology, syntax, semantics, pragmatics, and historical linguistics (*Webster's*, p. 1119).

Nursing is defined and described in various ways. Rogers (1980) described nursing as a science of unitary human beings and the art of "imaginative and creative use of this knowledge in human service" (p. 122). Peplau (1952) and Orem (1971) describe nursing as an interpersonal process. Boykin and Schoenhofer (1993) describe nursing as caring and a professional service "nurturing persons living caring and growing in caring" (p. 22). Meleis and Trangenstein in Meleis (1997) define nursing as "facilitating transitions to achieve a sense of well-being" (p. 118). Roach (1987) declares that in nursing, caring is unique since all the attributes that describe nursing have their origin in caring. Purnell and Locsin (2000) describe nursing as being generated and mediated by caring intentionality.

THE LANGUAGE OF NURSING: A DEFINITION

The language of nursing, therefore, may be understood and defined as a matrix of nursing caring intentionality expressed in a body of words and in gestures arising out of nursing's unique perspectives, knowledge base, and practice. Focused on the whole person, the language of nursing embeds and integrates other languages necessary to care for the whole person and to collaborate and communicate with others in that care. Nurses construct their language from out of their practice—days and nights of communicating in pithy, short stabs of terse phraseology, loaded with meaning and short with time to express caring. Language is also generated from nursing research and education as theory. Alternately, language used in nursing practice which is from the knowledge base and perspectives of *other* professions and disciplines may be described *not* as the language of nursing, but as language that is used in nursing.

PHILOSOPHICAL PERSPECTIVES ON LANGUAGE

Buber (1965) looks upon language not only as a means of communication, but also as the embodiment of meaning which resides in dialogue. According to Buber, dialogue is where we are turned to one another and present in the mutuality of inner action. Dialogue takes place when we perceive the other by *becoming aware*.

Buber posits that there are three ways in which we are able to perceive a living person with our eyes: Perceiving as an *observer* occurs when one is "wholly intent" (p. 8) in fixing the observed person in mind, and where the person is observed as a total of parts or traits. The observer probes and notes each part.

On the other hand, the *onlooker* pays no attention to parts but merely to an existence, and waits in openness to see what presents itself. Both observer and onlooker share their regard of the living person as an object, separated from themselves. These stances answer to the reductionist perspective of medicine and other disciplines where language-specific expressions focus on a person as being the sum of a number of parts.

In contrast with perception as an observer or onlooker, Buber (1965) addresses perceiving the other by *becoming aware*. Becoming aware is a subjective response to something that has spoken to one's own life; it is the response of inner speech. In nursing, specific philosophical understandings such as mutuality, intersubjectivity, and caring moment are examples of the rich nurse–patient relationship expressed in the language of nursing. These demonstrate the unitary concept of person as being more than the sum of parts and irreducible. In nursing, the concepts of "whole person" and "wholeness of person" (Boykin & Schoenhofer, 1993) express this idea.

Heidegger (1993), quoting Humboldt, describes the multidimensional nature of language as "the eternally self-repeating *labor of spirit* to make *articulated sound* capable of being an expression of thought" (p. 403), and later elaborates by saying, "We not only *speak* language, we speak *from out* of it" (p. 411); (emphases in original). According to both Heidegger (1993) and Buber (1965), language as embodied meaning is a vehicle for the spoken and unspoken, and thus for the expression of the inner person.

Merleau-Ponty (1962) offers the description that language is the "subject's taking up of a position in the world of his meanings" (p. 193), and is a "phonetic gesture" that modulates and coordinates experience between the speaker and listener. Van Manen (1990) describes an authentic speaker as a "true listener, able to attune to the deep tonalities of language that normally fall out of our accustomed way range of hearing" (p. 111). The understanding is implicate that the language of communication in nursing extends beyond mere representation through sound.

If the language of nursing, then, is a rich matrix arising out of nursing's unique knowledges and practice, how can this distinct language be regarded as a technology? Nurses use jargon, slang, and rich metaphors daily in their practice. How do expressions such as "frequent flyer" (a patient who is often hospitalized), "walkie-talkie" (a patient who needs minimal assistance), and "cabbage" (CABG, or coronary artery bypass graft) contribute to understanding the language of nursing as a technology?

THE LANGUAGE OF NURSING AS TECHNOLOGY

Overview

Technology has been described severally as drugs, medical devices, and procedures (Cram, Wheeler, & Lessard, 1995); as process, act, or action (Jones & Alexander, 1993); and as "people, tools, and techniques in organized systems of interactions to achieve human goals" (Bush, 1983, p. 36).

Heidegger (1993) refines the meaning of technology as a way of revealing and as "the name not only for the activities and skills of the craftsman, but also for the arts of the mind and the fine arts. *Techne* belongs to bringing-forth, to *poiesis*; it is something poetic" (p. 318).

Much has been written in the nursing literature about the language of nursing (Bjornsdottir, 1998; Carlson-Catalano, 1993; Casey & Hendricks, 1995; Crawford et al., 1999; David, 1995; Drevdahl, 1998; O'Brien & Pearson, 1993; Villaneuve, 1994). The use of imaginative and linguistic artifices such as the metaphor and figurative language has been extensively examined (Burke & Wilson, 1997; Cunningham, 1993; Froggatt, 1998; Hartrick & Schreiber, 1998; Hewison, 1997; Hiraki, 1998; Malone, 1999; Walker, 1997). Continuously evolving, the language of nursing is a dynamic organizing framework for achieving the goals of nursing. As a technology, nursing language exemplifies the idea of art in process, and language as action (Jones & Alexander, 1993). Technology is expressed as intentioned language revealing and communicating deliberate human interaction (Purnell & Locsin, 2000).

Contemporary professional nursing is grounded by an extensive nursing knowledge base. Scientific nursing research, increasingly accessible higher education, widening scope of clinical practice, and greater autonomy for nurses provide a context for the development of an increasingly complex, professional nursing language. Nurse scientists, theorists, and clinicians express their nursing in the succinct and dynamic language of nursing theory. The language of nursing theory itself guides and nurtures the perspective of the nurse. Expressing culture and compassion in linguistic artifice, the language of nursing reveals caring intention in the ideals of theory, the richness of metaphor, in context-driven slang and jargon, and in the languages of other professions and disciplines which are integrated into the nursing language matrix.

LANGUAGE "ON THE FLOOR"

Nursing practice is influenced and shaped by language (Bjornsdottir, 1998). When the language that nurses use does not reflect a nursing perspective, it affects nursing's model for practice (Carlson-Catalano, 1993). Language is used by nurses to create, organize, develop, enact, envision, and synthesize nursing beliefs, knowledge, values, and practice. Context-specific nursing language, such as professional jargon, is frequently learned and re-enforced during change of shift report, where seasoned nurses teach inexperienced nurses what it means to be a nurse (Wolf, 1989). Nurses display socialization by their ease with jargon and with abbreviations of commonly used terms, such as "fem pop" for femoral popliteal bypass and CA as a euphemism for cancer. Mastery of professional jargon contributes to acceptance as part of the team and to clinical proficiency perceived by others. The abbreviated, rapid-fire expression of nurses' linguistic shorthand in report is loaded with tacit knowing of nursing and medical interventions to be enacted with patients. These interventions are translated into context-specific jargon again and passed on in chain manner to nurses of the next shift.

Nurses often show "ownership" of patients in personalization of linguistic expressions. Such expressions as "He's going to code *on me*" or "He's getting 'tachy' *on me*" (experiencing tachycardia) are linguistic subtleties of speech which declare relationship and responsibility, and anticipate action. Nursing intention is revealed in languaging awareness and watchful concern. In the expression "on me," the locus of commitment is shown firmly seated in the nurse.

However, the evolution of nursing language as a technology is not limited to formalized theory or processes, or to linguistic devices such as jargon, slang, or metaphor. The roots of modern nursing language begin with Florence Nightingale, in the hospital nursing schools of the late nineteenth century.

NURSES' STORIES

Heidegger tapped into the compassion and beauty of nursing when he included in his understanding of technology "the arts of the mind and the fine arts . . . it is something poetic" (1993, p. 318). Nurses tell their stories not in the language of medical case presentation, nor the format of giving report, but in the caring, vulnerable expression of self. Nurses communicate their nursing caring in many ways, through oral and written story, through poetry, art, and music. Boykin and Schoenhofer (1991) propose story as a way to organize and communicate nursing knowledge. In nurses' stories, the lived relationship between the nurse and the one nursed is illuminated and brought to vivid life. Nurses share their knowledge in stories that are congruent with real life, and it is these stories which inspire, teach, encourage, and affirm. The following example is a nurse's story about a 40-year-old woman dying of cancer. The nurse was assisting another nurse with her patient "load" and saw the patient on this one occasion.

"I walked in the room and in her bed by the window, the patient lay comatose; pale, still, with only the rasp of her labored breathing breaking the silence. My eye followed the lines from her chest to a maze of connections; lines that led to IV poles, med pumps; line from her nasal cannula that connected to the humidifier and oxygen unit on the wall; the gentle background hissing of the suction pump with its coiled tubes, and a Foley tube from her body leading downwards to the empty bag that said her kidneys were no longer functioning.

In the corner of the room, backed against the wall, a man sat bolt upright, with arms folded defensively and with grim countenance. I introduced myself. He didn't respond verbally, but gave a brief nod of his head, so I proceeded to give meds via IV push. "What are you giving her?" he barked. After receiving an explanation, he retreated again into a brittle silence, crossed arms in a wall against his chest, intently surveying my every move across the chasm that separated him from his daughter.

Once the medication had infused into the central line, I paused, reflecting on the worn body of the woman before me. Feeling deep compassion for this soul who had suffered so much and who was soon to be going "home," I reached out and tenderly caressed her doll-like pink cheeks with the back of my hand, and smoothed out the lifeless stubs of yellow hair that were brittle against the pillow.

"What are you doing!" he barked once more, "taking her temperature?" "No," I replied, continuing to caress her face, "I am touching her heart." His face just seemed to crumple and with shoulders heaving and tears streaming down his cheeks, he raised his hands to his face and cried. She died the next day.

The rest of the story . . .

"It is so hard. It has been so long. Two years of fighting, and it has come to this. I can't do anything for her, can't even hold her. All I can do is sit here and watch her suffer. She can't last much longer. I don't know if I can."

I don't really know how long I spent with him. We were communicating with touch, and word, and look, and even in poignant silences. We talked openly about his daughter and her life, and how it was cut short. It was a brief review of her life, and, I think, the beginning of her father's farewell song. I took her father by the hand and led him over to the bed. As I held away the barriers of tubes, father and daughter were able to embrace, perhaps for the last time. I hope she could feel him—maybe she did, but I know that he could feel her, and that's what he needed to be able to let her go.

(Used with permission)

Nurses' stories are a link between practice and nursing's ontology and epistemology (Boykin & Schoenhofer, 1991). Nurses learn from each other through story. In nursing situations such as in the story above, the ontological reality and existence of nursing is located and affirmed. The link with epistemology becomes apparent in the ability of the nurse to reflect on the meaning in the words describing nursing in the situation and to learn from them. Nursing theories may be recalled which are appropriate for the phenomena taking place; new theories may be developed or existing theories in nursing and other disciplines may be investigated and even refuted; for example, anticipatory grief theory or bereavement stage theory (Kubler-Ross, 1968). The language used in nursing stories may include biomedical information, but the language matrix of nursing distinctly focuses on the whole person.

THE INFLUENCE OF OTHER DISCIPLINES

There are many pressures which affect the language that nurses use in daily practice. In the complex arena of health care, nurses are subject to the language and vocabulary of other professions and disciplines. Depending upon the area of practice, especially those incorporating high technology, nurses utilize, adapt, and adopt languages from disciplines such as medicine, psychology, engineering, and architecture in order to be able to communicate. With each different setting, nurses must accommodate and relearn meanings and implications of profession-driven languages in order to practice.

Other pressures exist which directly affect the language and practice of nursing. These pressures have their roots in society and in the place and evolution of women in the social order. In nursing, social pressures may be easily traced back over 100 years to the era of Florence Nightingale, when modern nursing began.

NURSING, SOCIETY, AND LANGUAGE: AN EVOLUTION

The reverence which is accorded Nightingale for her contribution to modern nursing is almost legendary. According to Reverby (1994), however, she contributed to some of the problems which faced American nursing at the end of the nineteenth century. Because of her beliefs about womanhood, Nightingale sought to organize a separate female nursing hierarchy which would supposedly share power in health care with male-dominated areas of medicine. The nurse work force was almost entirely women and remained so, and altruism and obedience to duty were demanded. With the exception of work in psychiatric hospitals, nursing was regarded as women's work by society, and by Nightingale herself (Reverby, 1994).

Nursing provided the opportunity for women to get outside of the home: "[The fact that] . . . nurses, as women without votes, husbands, money, or power in the 19th century United States, had established a separate occupation for women, formed alliances to control their lives and work, moved toward professional status, and were paid for their labors" (Baer, 1990, p. 26). Social changes which impacted the status of women also impacted language and values, and filtered into nursing practice and into the language of nursing. The language of nursing evolved slowly, concomitant with the emancipation and transformation of women from the status of maids and servants into professional nurses, educated and equipped to heal.

Accordingly, as the age of technology burgeoned in the twentieth century, the nurse who was used to dodging mud puddles in long, floor-length, modest dresses in the nineteenth century became the streamlined nurse who served in battlefields and wore pants. The language of the nurturing, motherly nurse became studded with medical phrases as nurses became increasingly more responsible for handling technological advances of the era.

GENDER AND LANGUAGE IN NURSING

Then . . . A Time Capsule

At the rate of about two or three per week toward the end of the nineteenth century, American hospitals were established by male physicians *in order to offer nursing care by women* (Ashley, 1976). In the first decade of the twentieth century, 1,851 new hospitals were established. Women served essentially as indentured servants in exchange for their "training" and were expected to assist the physicians in their work and answer to the hospitals' needs (Ashley, 1976).

In 1886, the graduating class of the Boston Training School for Nurses was addressed by a physician. "The doctor is always right," Dr. William Richardson said. "Always be loyal to the physician," he added, warning nurses not to be "tempted" to impress the doctor with their knowledge because "what error could be more stupid?" (Luck & Kellman, 1983, p. 244). Dr. Richardson was well aware that the course of study in most medical schools was more limited than that found in many nursing schools (Ashley, 1976).

In 1924, the American Medical Association (AMA) declared that the nurse's duty was to care for patients under the supervision of a physician. Paternalistically, and in order to maintain power and control over nurses training in hospitals as a source of profits, the AMA changed the name of its Council on Medical Education to "The Council on Medical Education *and Hospitals*." By doing so, the AMA set itself up as the authority on nursing and over nursing, and ignored the female-organized Society of Training School Superintendents. This organization of nursing educators was to later become the National League of Nursing Education.

Now ...

As recently as 1970, a position statement of the AMA declared that the "logical place" of nurses is at the physician's side in order to "extend the hands of the physician" (1970, p. 1882). Arising out of tradition and social constraints, biomedical discourse continues to be enframed in male-gendered language. In the highly structured medical environment of contemporary Western hospitals, the volatile issue of gender inequities has been carefully held in abeyance. Ashley (1976) succinctly notes, however, that "Sex-defined roles have always been, and still are, the most outstanding characteristic division of labor within hospitals" (p. 18). A cursory examination of any health care institution will confirm that 100 years after Nightingale, the power structure in health care institutions is relatively unchanged: Nurses are still predominantly female, and physicians are still predominantly male. Boards of Nursing still retain within their ranks physicians to "oversee" nursing licensure exams. Licensure exams themselves constitute medical procedures in which physicians no longer care to be directly involved, and which symbolize control retained by medicine. Physicians in such positions of authority over nurses and nursing knowledge legitimize and sanction proliferation of the medical perspective, language, and philosophy as exemplars in an exam to test nursing practice.

In practice, physicians are seldom present to see the effects of the medical interventions they prescribe; absentee "supervision" is the norm. It is accepted as "nursing's job" to perform many medical tasks, to monitor their effects, and then to report back to the physician. Nurses are thus rated on their ability to be physician "helpers," and conditioned to regard their nursing knowledge and language as being of lesser value.

Hospital "nursing" competencies, while undoubtedly fulfilling a much needed role in contemporary hospital nursing, lay claim once again to the idea that nurses expert in technological use and interpretation are the medical "ideal" since the physician's physical presence is not needed, merely his "oversight." Communication becomes more and more immersed in linguistic patterns of medical expression, so that mastery of medical language becomes a badge of expertise and a measure of social rank within an oppressed group such as nursing (Roberts, 1983).

The Female "Voice"

The most casual observer cannot help but see the web of sociohistorical entanglement between nursing, medicine, and the issue of gender-motivated behavior and language. Gilligan (1993) illuminates the loss and stifling of the female voice, and the perpetuation of "a male-voiced civilization and an order of living that is founded on disconnection from women" (p. xi). She describes voice as being "the core of self," and "composed of breath and sound, words, rhythm, and language" (p. xvi). It is evident that throughout the complex development of nursing as a distinct discipline, nurses have been subject to societal forces that have restricted and disallowed the essentiality of female relational exchange as a valid form of communication in a male-dominated medical system: "the capacity for autonomous thinking, clear decision-making, and responsible action—are those associated with masculinity and considered undesirable as attributes of the feminine self" (Gilligan, 1982, p. 17). Nurses have been compelled not only to speak the language of medicine in order to advance in their profession, but to act and socialize into a male-dominated and -socialized system.

However, while argument may be made concerning the suppression of the female voice and of its lack of formal acceptance in contemporary nursing, balanced consideration must also be given to expression of the male voice in nursing. To imply that only female nurses are sensitive, caring, expressive individuals is to endorse the same gender differentiation in nursing that was espoused a century ago. Regardless of gender, culture, and generation, nurses communicate their nursing in the language of nursing; that is, in the matrix of inherited, scientific, and contemporary nursing knowledge. The language of caring intention in nursing is *genderless*.

INFLUENCE OF TECHNOLOGIES ON NURSING LANGUAGE

The advent of the electronic age and the integration of computer technology into health care has produced a radical change in the ways that nurses think, talk about, and record their practice. Nurses' communications have been gradually pressured to accommodate and record use and outcomes of the growing array of biomedical technologies, ranging from the introduction of the use of the physician's stethoscope to the current, unprecedented and unrivaled creation of electronic medical diagnostic and practice technologies. The intense research, rapid advancement, and use of life-enhancing pharmaceutical products also influenced language, so that no patient is without some form of medical technology, even in the home. Hiraki (1998) notes that corporate metaphorical language has intruded into the language of home health nurses and systematically distorts meaning and communication. For example, a health plan member is no longer a patient, or a client, or even a consumer of health care, but is instead a customer. Nurses accept, integrate, and communicate among themselves and with patients, in the adopted languages of medicine, sociology, psychology, engineering, and other disciplines, as well as their own; however, according to Hiraki (1998), nursing's discourse about its own practice is marginalized.

Charting

It may be observed that the language of nursing has been substantially eliminated from patient charts and records, and has been supplanted by the business language of managed care. A dichotomy exists. Nurses use a language of rationale and objectivity to communicate about their patients with medicine and other professions, and a language of intense, focused relationship to communicate with their patients and among themselves. Nursing language routinely recorded in practice is rapidly becoming extinct: Handwritten nursing "notes" and care plans have given way to check-off boxes on a computer screen. The uniqueness of nursing communications has been standardized into a language and format that a computer can use for data and the living patient is reduced to bytes of information. Few nurses prefer hand charting after being familiarized with computer charting menus. Recording nursing interventions and outcomes is simplified in a check-off system and more easily adapted to the "swinging door" of rapid admissions and discharges in acute care institutions. Ironically, it was Nightingale who first suggested, in 1860, "If you find it helps you to note down such things on a bit of paper, in pencil, by all means do so" (Nightingale, 1969, p. 112).

NURSING INFORMATICS—THE "NEW" LANGUAGE OF NURSING

While the nursing literature abounds in discussion of what constitutes the language of nursing, cries are even so being heard for a "new" language which all professions can understand. What becomes apparent in collaborative consideration of a "new" language are the "new" non-nurse users with a vested interest in a specialized form of communication: interfacing health care disciplines, a vast array of human and technological support systems, the hospital and home health industry, and managed care.

Perhaps the most profound influence on the way nursing will be understood and practiced in the new century is the now ubiquitous corporate concept of "managed care" in which nurses remain key providers of information concerning patient health and patient care. The health care industry not only assiduously seeks every datum of that information from nursing, but demands it be supplied in formats and systems which efficiently answer to their unit/cost focus, yet fail egregiously to serve the human needs and focus of the patient and nurse. The allure of technology, of its speed, clarity, and ease of use, appears to offer a way out of the burdens created by corporate metaphors of downsizing and right-sizing. It is routinely recognized that computer technology requires dedicated maintenance personnel and support systems. However, nursing itself may also be seen as a tacit support system of computer technology in its provision of data to be processed: The technology is provided with a reason for being. The language of nursing is steadily being segmented and substituted by a "computer-friendly" language of reductionism in order to be acceptable as computer data.

Institutional demands facilitate the intrusion of language and meaning of non-health-related disciplines into the language of nursing. Multifactorial specifics such as "skill mix" and "engineered" give new meaning to the idea of quality of nursing services. Prompted and pushed by investors' "bottom line" financial priorities, the movement within the discipline of nursing is toward a "standard" language of nursing with common nursing diagnoses, interventions, and outcomes language. This standard language will be "engineered" to readily convert to reductive, interdisciplinary computer databases and accommodate institutional and global requirements. Snyder, Egan, and Nojima (1996) suggest that the lack of a common intervention language will adversely affect international collaboration. Several questions arise: What will be the purpose of the collaboration? Who will benefit from the international collaboration of shared data? Will the patient benefit who has already been reduced to data?

NURSING—A MATTER OF HUMAN VALUES

Regardless of the language spoken and of the culture in which nursing caring is communicated, the matrix of nursing language stands uniquely as a technology of caring. Arising out of practice, research, and education, nursing language mediates intentionality and expression and is communicated in expressions and ways that are peculiar to the culture, institution, or global venue. The perpetuation of nursing values is achieved through its language and transmitted from human to human. The language of nursing caring is the foundational matrix upon which all other communications and languages rest and derive their value.

REFERENCES

American Medical Association. (1970). Position Statement. *Journal of the American Medical Association*.

Anspach, R. R. (1994). The language of case presentation. In P. Conrad & R. Kern (Eds.), *The sociology of health & illness: Critical perspectives* (pp. 312–331). New York: St. Martin's Press.

Ashley, J. A. (1976). *Hospitals, paternalism, and the role of the nurse.* New York: Teachers College Press.

Baer, E. D. (1990). Editor's notes. *Nursing in America: A history of social reform* [Video]. New York: National League for Nursing.

Bjornsdottir, K. (1998). Language, ideology, and nursing practice. *Scholarly Inquiry for Nursing Practice: An International Journal, 12*(4), 347–361.

Boykin, A., & Schoenhofer, S. (1991). Story as link between nursing practice, ontology, epistemology. *Image: Journal of Nursing Scholarship, 23*(4), 245–248.

Boykin, A., & Schoenhofer, S. (1993). *Nursing as caring: A model for transforming practice.* New York: National League for Nursing Press.

Buber, M. (1965). *Between man and man.* New York: Macmillan.

Burke, L. M., & Wilson, A. (1997). Mental models, metaphors and their use in the education of nurses. *Journal of Nursing Management, 5*(6), 351–357.

Burkhart, L. (1997, Spring–Summer). Nursing standardized language to promote professionalism. *Perspectives in Parish Nursing Practice, 1,* 3, 11.

Carlson-Catalano, J. (1993). What is the language of nursing? *Nursing Forum, 28*(4), 22–26.

Casey, M., & Hendricks, J. (1995). Nursing diagnosis: Language antithetical to nursing's ontology. *Contemporary Nurse, 4*(3), 107–112.

Cram, N., Wheeler, J., & Lessard, C. (1995). Ethical issues of life-sustaining technology. *IEEE Technology and Society Magazine, 14*(1), 21–28.

Crawford, P., Johnson, A., Brown, B., & Nolan, P. (1999). The language of mental health nursing reports: Firing paper bullets? *Journal of Advanced Nursing, 29*(2), 331–340.

Cunningham, N. (1993). Identity, metaphors, and power. *Clinical Issues in Perinatal Women's Health, 4*(4), 634–640.

David, N. (1995). Language of primary nursing. *Elderly Care, 7*(2), 15–17.

Drevdahl, E. (1998). Diamond necklaces: Perspectives on power and the language of "community." *Scholarly Inquiry for Nursing Practice: An International Journal, 12*(4), 303–317.

Froggatt, K. (1998). The place of metaphor and language in exploring nurses' emotional work. *Journal of Advanced Nursing, 28*(2), 332–338.

Gilligan, C. (1993). *In a different voice: Psychological theory and women's development.* Cambridge, MA: Harvard University Press.

Hartrick, G., & Schreiber, R. (1998). Imaging ourselves: Nurses' metaphors of practice. *Journal of Holistic Nursing, 16*(4), 420–434.

Heidegger, M. (1971). *Poetry, language, thought.* New York: Harper and Row.

Heidegger, M. (1993). *Basic writings.* San Francisco: HarperCollins.

Hewison, A. (1997). The language of management: An enduring challenge. *Journal of Nursing Management, 5*(3), 133–141.

Hiraki, A. (1998). Corporate language and nursing practice. *Nursing Outlook, 46,* 115–119.

Jones, C., & Alexander, J. (1993). The technology of caring: A synthesis of technology and caring for nursing administration. *Nursing Administration Quarterly, 17*(2), 11–20.

Kubler-Ross, E. (1968). *On death and dying.* New York: Macmillan.

Luck, S., & Kellman, S. (1983). A quiet revolution: Holistic nursing. *Whole Life Times* (reprint), 244–248.

Malone, R. E. (1999). Policy as product: Morality and metaphor in health policy discourse. *Hastings Center Report, 29*(3), 16–22.

Meleis, A. I. (1997). *Theoretical nursing: Development and progress* (3rd ed.). Philadelphia: Lippincott.

Merleau-Ponty, M. (1962). *Phenomenology of perception*. New York: Routledge.

Nightingale, F. (1969). *Notes on nursing: What it is and what it is not*. New York: Dover Publications.

O'Brien, B., & Pearson, A. (1993). Unwritten knowledge in nursing: Consider the spoken as well as the written word. *Scholarly Inquiry for Nursing Practice: An International Journal, 7*(2), 111–127.

Orem, D. (1971). *Nursing: Concepts of practice*. New York: McGraw-Hill.

Peplau, H. E. (1952). *Interpersonal relations, differences, and relations* (reprint 1991). New York: Springer.

Purnell, M., & Locsin, R. (2000). *Intentionality: Unification in nursing*. Manuscript submitted for publication.

Reverby, S. (1994). A caring dilemma: Womanhood and nursing in historical perspective. In P. Conrad & R. Kern (Eds.), *The sociology of health & illness: Critical perspectives* (pp. 210–221). New York: St. Martin's Press.

Ricoeur, P. (1992). *Oneself as another*. Chicago: University of Chicago Press.

Roach, S. (1987). *The human act of caring*. Ottawa: Canadian Hospital Association.

Roberts, S. J. (1983). Oppressed group behavior: Implications for nursing. *Advances in Nursing Science, 5*(3), 21–30.

Rogers, M. (1980). *The science of unitary man* [audiotapes]. New York: Media for Nursing.

Snyder, M., Egan, E., & Nojima, Y. (1996). Defining nursing interventions. *Image: Journal of Nursing Scholarship, 28*(2), 137–141.

Van Manen, M. (1990). *Researching lived experience*. Albany: State University of New York Press.

Villaneuve, M. J. (1994). Recruiting and retaining men in nursing: A review of the literature. *Journal of Professional Nursing, 10*(4), 217–228.

Walker, C. A. (1997). Imagination, metaphor and nursing theory. *Journal of Theory Construction and Testing, 1*(1), 22–27.

Webster's Encyclopedic Unabridged Dictionary (1996). New York: Gramercy Books.

Wolf, Z. R. (1989). Learning the professional jargon of nursing during change of shift report. *Holistic Nursing Practice, 4*(1), 78–83.

Chapter 6

Technology, De-skilling, and Nurses: The Impact of the Technologically Changing Environment

Ruth G. Rinard

INTRODUCTION

A recent National Public Radio broadcast on the impact of the Internet interviewed an enthusiast who foresaw more equality, democracy, and individual expression. A more cautious voice, Susan Douglas, of the University of Michigan, reminded the audience that such claims at the beginning of the radio era were quickly eclipsed by mass network broadcasting. Since World War II, the nursing environment has experienced several distinct waves of technological change. Internal histories of the nursing profession have seen technological change as a story of new roles, increasing education, and a research-based, scientific nursing practice. More attention to the broader social and cultural landscape reveals another story. It is the story of the fragmentation, of de-skilling of nursing, and the reproduction and recreation of gendered jobs and social relationships in the capitalistic health care environment.

Theoretical Concerns

Understanding the impact of technology on nursing requires concepts from the history of technology, from labor process theory, and from gender studies. First, technology is not confined to machines. It includes change at the site of production, the transfer of production between workstations and their coordination. The dramatic increase in numbers and types of drugs is similar to the introduction of machines, specialized care units similar to batch processing, and critical care information pathways similar to automated manufacturing.

Second, the introduction of technologies is not determined by their rationality or cost-effectiveness alone, but also by social relations or government largesse which favors a particular direction (Smith, 1977; Noble, 1984). While technologies have a material base, their meaning, use, and skill valuations are determined historically by cultural and social forces rather than simply material (Cocburn, 1983).

Third, within a Marxian analysis of capitalism, the labor process re-creates the social relationships of production even as new technologies are introduced. Harry Bravermann (1974) has argued that the introduction of mechanization, automation, and modern management techniques led to a de-skilling of work. Wagner (1980) applied these ideas to the rise of hospital nursing showing how de-skilling occurred. Michael Burawoy, in *Manufacturing Consent* (1979), critiqued and extended these ideas, showing how workers accepted de-skilling to gain relative satisfaction in the game of making it on the shop floor and thereby obscured the expropriation of unpaid labor. The internal labor market, he argued, diffused resentment toward management and redirected it toward co-workers.

Fourth, gender studies suggest that skills, particularly those tacit skills acquired by women *qua* women in their domestic and social lives outside the workplace, are gendered (Melosb, 1982; Reverby, 1987; West, 1982). Such skills may be particularly vulnerable as new technologies emerge (Benson, 1986; Wood, 1982). Finally, management may utilize gender constructions in the wider culture to secure acquiescence to de-skilling (Sturdy, 1992).

METHODS

A current analysis of the *American Journal of Nursing*, the first and foremost nursing journal in the postwar period, was undertaken in five-year intervals. The content examined included advertisements and recruitment notices as well as published articles and regular departments. Changes were noted in the types of articles, in the introduction of new departments, and in the changing character and appeal of advertisements and recruitment notices. On the basis of this content analysis, a rough periodization was constructed. The first period, from 1950 to 1960, was characterized by the introduction of mechanical techniques and a myriad of new drugs. A second period, from 1965 to 1980, saw the introduction of electronic machinery and specialized care units. The third period, from 1980 to the present, introduced technologies to control, streamline, and predict care. Each of these will be discussed in turn.

RESULTS

1950–1960

Postwar fascination with technology found its way into the pages of the *American Journal of Nursing*. Plexitron drip chambers produced atomic bomb–like "flashballs" when squeezed (*American Journal of Nursing*, 1955d). But the threat of the Cold War also led to American Medical Association (AMA) advertisements against national health insurance as socialized medicine. Social roles narrowed. Good personal adjustment and the absence of conflict became synonymous with good nursing. In the move to suburbia and childbearing, nurses, like other women, were targeted by *Journal* ads as consumers of new products—frozen orange juice, Gerber's baby food, cellophane tape, and Dacron uniforms.

New medicines were the new technology. In 1950, medicine ads were confined to Dermassage, Desitin, Riasoll for psoriasis, and baby formula. By 1955, ads for penicillin, ilotyan (*American Journal of Nursing*, 1955a), archromycin with its "special dropper to measure each dose quickly" (*American Journal of Nursing*, 1955b) competed with tetracycline and terramycin for the nurse's attention. Reserpine and chlorpromazine, new psycho-active drugs, promised to transform mental hospitals.

Intravenous fluids became widely used (Anderson, 1955). Venipuncture, not appropriate for nurses, was started by doctors or residents. Nurses managed the large quantities used—1,000 cc over four hours, 3,000 cc over eight hours—using carts with supplies for eight to ten patients. Nurses spend much of the shift starting, stopping, and adjusting these rapid infusions.

Blood products—albumin, fibrinogen, and gamma globulin—became available in 1955, drastically changing the labor process. A patient might be given 20–30 transfusions as protein for body repair over several days (Crews, 1955). Electric call bells, pneumatic tubes, and intercoms changed nurses' relationships with patients and hospital departments. Penicillin, frequently given IM every two hours, increased time spent sterilizing and re-sharpening needles. Each unit now had an autoclave to tend (Edelson, 1955). Oxygen from wall units went to incubators, new equipment for "convenient infant care" (*American Journal of Nursing*, 1955c).

In response to the separation of tasks entailed in these technological changes, one nurse wrote, "The assignment . . . make(s) the average nurse more a robot than a woman. This system puts nursing on the factory level" (*American Journal of Nursing*, 1950a). Another wondered "If the patient has the feeling . . . that he is on an assemble line?" (*American Journal of Nursing*, 1950b). Lamenting the loss, another wrote, "These is something tragic in a nurse (who) . . . resembles a player-piano-mechanically perfect, but without passion, anyone can master skills, but nursing is a vocation" (*American Journal of Nursing*, 1955d). The sense of loss was connected to the decline of direct personal bodily care (Lesser & Kearns, 1955). Pictures portraying "oxygen in every room," "plenty of antibiotics," and "new and greater x-rays" were dismissed with the caption "But what is the state of the patient's back so long as he lies in bed?" (*American Journal of Nursing*, 1950c, p. 34).

How did nursing leaders respond to the dilemmas posed by technical changes? If old craft traditions and tacit skills learned by women as women in their roles in the family and the community were being undermined, perhaps it was possible to reclaim them by objectifying them in the language of social science. The skills of talking with patients were emphasized (Peplau, 1960). An editorial asserted, "We believe that the application of social skills is the essential part of professional nursing. As nursing moved into higher education, differentiation between a "technical" and a "professional" nurse depended on the ability to discuss tacit skills in social science jargon. In the process, technical skills were devalued. Nursing leaders believed that naming tacit skills in academic language conferred an objective reality to those skills which could forestall changes in the labor process created by the new technology.

1965–1980

In the 1960s and 1970s, new nursing environments were created by a different sort of technological change, the organization to specialized care units. Machines of all kinds—dialysis units, cardiac monitors, fetal monitoring, and automatic recording devices were associated with the development of these units. The editorial for the one issue with articles on technology declared, "If the nurse has an uneasy feeling about today's wondrous machines, some of which seem to be encroaching on her practice, she's not much different from other people. Much as it is natural to resist them, we'll have to get used to them because they're here" (*American Journal of Nursing*, 1965, p. 67). Some thought the significance of the recording machines lay in reduced disputes with physicians. "The nurse and the physician can ascertain simultaneously . . . the vital signs" (George, 1965, p. 68). Others marveled at the degree of individual variation the machine revealed. Still others saw more clearly that the new machines required new learning and new responsibility (Imboden & Wynn, 1965). Dialysis nurses pointed in this direction by talking of "technical nursing observation" skills (Tsurk, 1965). A few writers even spoke of the creative uncertainty within limits that the new machines afforded as an antidote to the de-skilled drudgery of most nursing work. But this view was editorially dismissed. "Today's machines, especially electronic ones, are forcing us to see machines in a new perspective. Since we [can't] be expected to be experts in electrical engineering, we have no [choice] but to leave that to others and keep our focus on the patient to which the machine is attached" (*American Journal of Nursing*, 1965, p. 67).

Although the official view in the journal left no room for new valuations of skills, ads and letters spoke to the pervasive reality of technological change. One Pacquins ad from 1965 was particularly striking. All previous Pacquins ads showed gracefully draped, polished, ring-adorned hands. But this one showed unpolished hands holding a syringe ready for an injection. Earlier recruitment ads had stressed new equipment or new surgical suites as belonging to the hospital. Now recruitment ads emphasized special technical skills belonging to the individual nurse. Letters give evidence of increased conflict between nurses around workplace-generated valuation of skill. One letter writer snidely remarked, "Knowledge of family and community will be lost in the pursuit of higher knowledge that says—this is an inverted T wave." (*American Journal of Nursing*, 1970, p. 246). The period from 1965 to 1980 saw the creation of highly technical new work environments, but also a studied refusal to look seriously at them. This refusal, it seems, was grounded in the belief that objective skills had already been defined and that feminine nature left no room for other new skill valuations.

1980–1990

The technological changes in this period involved attempts to control, streamline, and predict care. They ranged from institution-wide, computerized information systems, to novel organizational structures, to linkages between segments within health care. These technological changes, spurred by governmentally imposed cost-control measures, are still in progress. There were a few scattered references to early HMOs as news items, but no discussion of their implications for the labor process of nursing. What was more apparent in the pages of the *Journal* was the cost of the disjunction between the social scientific attempt to describe tacit skills and the real environment of the labor process. A letter writer complained that she was a "coma specialist" performing automatic, unconscious tasks (Pillette, 1980). Still another called herself an "artificial nurse." "You want to assess and plan and meet psycho-social needs," she wrote, "and this is what you get in a shift—checking IV's, refusing meds, O masks, pain shots, housekeeping stuff and dealing with docs" (Pope, 1975, p. 248). Yet an article on stress in nursing did not explore causes in the technological changes affecting the work environment itself, but offered tips on "how to make it work for you" through jogging, relaxation exercises, and expression of feelings (Scully, 1980, p. 913).

The story of the impact of technological change on nursing from 1950 to 1990 is thus a story of de-skilling. The introduction of new machines and equipment, of specialized care units and electronic monitoring, and the transformation of nursing by information system technology has and continues to radically alter daily routines of nurses. This change was experienced by nurses as a de-skilling in the Bravermannian sense. The tacit empathetic and relational skills which had been acquired in the process of forming a culturally acceptable feminine identity were difficult to articulate. This is also a transitional period in the larger society as women, on the one hand, are urged to think beyond traditional social role self-concepts, and, on the other hand, are encouraged to retain "natural, womanly characteristics" (e.g., bring home the bacon and cook it up in a pan, etc.). Nevertheless, their objectification in the language of social science did not render them less gendered. What was more apparent in the pages of the *Journal* was the cost of the disjunction between the social scientific attempt to describe tacit skills and the real environment of the labor process. An editorial proclaimed that "nursing is coming into its own," but acknowledged gendered aspects. Furthermore, the fact of naming these socially constructed, tacit skills made it more difficult for nurses either to see or to value other skills introduced or demanded by technological change.

Only as the hold of feminine cultural identity loosened in the 1970s, and wider models became possible were nurses able to acknowledge, and in some cases even value for themselves, new technical skills. But since, as we have argued, skills are not primarily objective categories, but a system of socially valued activities and attributes, glimmering recognition of new skills by nurses themselves was not enough.

Many of the new technological skills had formerly been the exclusive province of the largely male medical staff. As they crossed gender lines, these skills became devalued, merely technical things which anyone with a little training could do. The feminine cultural traits of patience, observation, and orderliness were now attached to the very same tasks, and the task itself became transformed into one suitable for women.

But the cultural valuation of technological innovation also played a significant role. Once a technological procedure was removed from the realm of novelty and performed more routinely, it became less interesting, even dull. It was no longer a cutting-edge skill. Even when it was apparent, in the 1980s and 1990s, that the naive, optimistic faith in technology of the 1950s was no longer viable and that technology had created unanticipated problems, solutions proposed by nurses were regarded not as valued innovations, but as part of the march of progress. These innovations were viewed as minor tinkering, and when practical solutions to human predicaments relied on relational skills to discern distress, to comfort, and to motivate patients caught up in complicated medical procedures, they were evaluated on both technological and gender grounds.

Against the technology-cum-gender skills landscape, nursing activities continued to be less valued on both counts.

IMPLICATIONS FOR THE FUTURE

The story of the changes in the work environment for nurses caused by the successive waves of technological change from 1950 to 1990 has implications for nursing as it continues to confront technological change. The major implication is that a logico-positivistic view of knowledge and skills has limited flexible responses to changed work environments. First, this framework assumed that the content of tacit knowledge can be fully objectified. Second, the professional legitimation of nursing through social science research was simply too narrow a part of cultural discourse to provide the hoped-for result. Third, the belief that nursing skill had been objectified, which has fostered the positivistic assumptions about knowledge, prevented a serious examination of technological change. Finally, the positivistic stance toward knowledge, accelerated by nursing's move to the academy in the 1960s, resulted in a static view of feminine nature. It could not be conceptualized as a more fluid social entity that might have provided nursing with more flexible responses to technological change. The larger perspective holds promise for giving us the understanding and flexibility to deal with continuing, technologically produced changes in our environment.

REFERENCES

Advertisement. (1950a). *American Journal of Nursing, 50*(1), 4.
Advertisement. (1950b). *American Journal of Nursing. 50*(6), 258.
Advertisement. (1950c). *American Journal of Nursing, 50*(9), 34.
Advertisement. (1955a). *American Journal of Nursing, 55*(1), 32.
Advertisement. (1955b). *American Journal of Nursing, 55*(2), 137.
Advertisement. (1955c). *American Journal of Nursing, 55*(2), 219.
Advertisement. (1955d). *American Journal of Nursing, 55*(4), 514.
Anderson, B. (1955). Nursing service and the law. *American Journal of Nursing, 55*(4), 438–439.
Benson, S. (1986). *Counter cultures: Saleswomen, managers, and customers in American department stores, 1890–1960.* Urbana: University of Illinois Press.
Bravermann, H. (1974). *Labor and monopoly capital: The degradation of work in the twentieth century.* New York: Monthly Review Press.
Burawoy, M. (1979). *Manufacturing consent.* Chicago: University of Chicago Press.
Cocburn, C. (1983). *Brothers: Male dominance and technological change.* London: Pluto Press.
Crews, H. (1955). Small hospital blood bank. *American Journal of Nursing, 55*(3), 320–321.

Edelson, R. (1955). Organizing the nursing service for a new hospital. *American Journal of Nursing, 55*(2), 198–201.

Editorial. (1965). *American Journal of Nursing, 65*(2), 67.

Editorial. (1970). *American Journal of Nursing, 70*(2), 246.

George, J. (1965). Electronic monitoring of vital signs. *American Journal of Nursing, 65*(2), 68–71.

Imboden, C., and Wynn, J. (1965). Coronary care area. *American Journal of Nursing, 65*(2), 72–76.

Knights, D., & Willmott, H. (1986). *Gender and the labour process.* Brookfield, VT: Gower.

Lesser, N., & Kearns, V. (1955). Nursing and bodily care. *American Journal of Nursing, 55*(6), 804–806.

Letter. (1955). *American Journal of Nursing, 55*(3), 260.

Melosh, B. (1982). *The physician's hand: Work culture and conflict in American nursing.* Philadelphia: Temple University Press.

Noble, D. (1984). *Forces of production: A social history of automation.* New York: Knopf.

Peplau, H. (1960). Talking with patients. *American Journal of Nursing, 60*(6), 964–966.

Pillette, P. (1980). Caution: Objectivity and specialization may be hazardous to your health. *American Journal of Nursing, 80*(9), 1588–1590.

Pope, N. (1975). Thoughts from an artificial nurse. *American Journal of Nursing, 75*, 248–249.

Reverby, S. (1987). *Ordered to care.* Cambridge: Cambridge University Press.

Scully, R. (1980). Stress in the nurse. *American Journal of Nursing, 80*, 912–917.

Smith, M. (1977). *Harper's Ferry and the new technology.* Ithaca, NY: Cornell University Press.

Sturdy, A. (1992). *Skill and consent.* London: Routledge.

Tsurk, C. (1965). Hemodialysis for acute renal failure. *American Journal of Nursing, 65*(2), 80–85.

Wagner, D. (1980). The proletarianization of nursing in the United States, 1932–1946. *International Journal of the Health Sciences, 10*, 271–290.

West, J. (1982). *Work, women, and the labour market.* London: Routledge.

Wood, S. (1982). *The degradation of work? Skill, deskilling and the labour process.* London: Hutchinson.

Part II

Practice Issues: Outcomes of Caring in Nursing

Chapter 7

Outcomes of Caring in High-Technology Practice Environments

Savina O. Schoenhofer

INTRODUCTION

As the world of health care moves to a concern with fiscal viability, the nursing profession is paying more and more attention to outcomes of care. Considerable effort has been put into the development of laborious and complicated taxonomies of nursing outcomes. A close study of these efforts reveals certain underlying assumptions, such as viewing nursing as an adjunct to medical treatment, with only token attempts to incorporate views of care based on nursing theory. The language systems used are clearly medical derivatives. The emphasis is largely on cost-related indicators such as treatment days, readmission rates, and time factors. In facilitating the understanding of outcomes from a nursing perspective, rather than from the traditional biomedical view, the following reflective exercise is suggested. The reader is invited to pause.

- Recollect a personal nursing situation that occurred in a technologically dependent environment that was a situation in which you felt you were truly nursing in the fullest sense.
- Reflect for a few moments, reliving the experience—people, objects, sights, sounds, smells, feelings. You may wish to write or record the story of this nursing situation for further reflection.
- What made this a situation in which you felt you were truly nursing? Describe the beauty of the situation in a sentence that begins with the words, "Nursing is . . ." What you have called into awareness and described captures the essence of what nursing means to you.

• Now recall or review a nursing outcomes system, perhaps one that is used at your employment setting. Does this system convey the beauty of your gift of nursing? Does it portray the real value of your nursing care—to your patient? To the health care institution? To the community? To your sense of yourself as nurse? Probably not.

Rather than illuminating the value of the nursing contribution to patient care, outcome taxonomies tend to obscure that which you and your patient find most valuable in your nursing.

ACCOUNTABILITY

The concept of accountability became a permanent fixture of the nursing lexicon during the consumerism era of the 1970s. Whatever altruistic motives made the concept attractive to nurses at that time, it is accountability that has come to signify fiscal responsibility. Accounting principles are used to interpret the value of nursing. It is no coincidence that subdivisions of nursing services are now widely called "cost centers." The language of economics has joined the language of medicine as the most commonly understood language of nursing. Practicing nurses do not need to be reminded that their service is primarily interpreted and evaluated in economic terms—we live with it and participate in it every day.

Accounting may be defined as an information system focused on the economic activities of an entity (Fess, Warren, & Reeve, 1993). The process of accounting involves analyzing, organizing, and recording transactions as income and expenditure categories, assigning monetary value to the analysis and summarizing the results of analysis meaningfully. This process describes the use of outcomes of nursing care. But what does it communicate about the real value of nursing? Any person who is highly skilled in the application of biomedical technologies can successfully contribute to the aims of the medical care of patients—witness the growing pressure to introduce "registered care technicians" (RCTs) into care settings as substitutes for nurses.

If nurses believe there is something special that nursing brings to patients, they must be able to bring knowledge of that "something special" from a tacit level to an explicit one. Nurses, particularly in expensive, high-technology settings, need to be able and willing to speak the language of nursing. Nurses have readily adopted the expectation that they acquire the ability to understand and communicate in other languages (e.g., medicine, economics), but have been reluctant to hold other health team members to a similar expectation regarding knowledge and skills in nursing language. When health care records and interdisciplinary team discussions focus only on the requirements and benefits of biomedical and economic implications of health care, nursing is not only undervalued, it is invisible—except as an adjunct to medicine and economics.

If nursing accountability does not reside in the realm of medicine and economics, what is its meaning in nursing? If outcomes of nursing care are not captured in patient days, readmission rates, and time factors, what are outcomes of nursing care? Without a clear, supportable, and articulated understanding of nurses' contributions to patient outcomes, why should nursing care be seen as anything other than support for medical care plans and health care efficiency models? Is it possible that well-trained RCTs are indeed adequate substitutes for nurses?

THE LANGUAGE OF NURSING

The language of nursing, as with any language, is an expression of the values, assumptions, and practices of members of the culture. The reader is invited to return to the remembered beautiful experience of nursing. There is the language of nursing! Now think for a moment about how this nursing situation was communicated formally, in the chart, in report, in rounds. What language system was used? Was it nursing or was it translated into another language, losing much of its meaning as nursing?

The language of nursing is, like its practice, personal. It involves words like caring, being with, connectedness, trust, courage, hope, humility, sharing, joy, suffering. Twentieth-century efforts to improve the professional status of nursing may have contributed to the "underground" character of the language of nursing. Nurses in practice roles and in roles focused on research and theory development have struggled to "transcend" the personal meaning of nursing in an effort to gain standing with disciplines whose contributions are more impersonal, rational, technological. Meanwhile, there is universal recognition that health care has become depersonalized, mechanical, and "bottom line" oriented. The language of nursing is missing and thus much of the potentially humanizing influence of nursing is also unrealized.

OUTCOMES OF NURSING CARE IN HIGH-TECHNOLOGY ENVIRONMENTS

The prevalent notion of outcomes derives from production concepts, inputting raw materials through the application of well-defined procedures to create a pre-envisioned, uniform end product that solves a pre-specified problem. The focus on patient compliance is an obvious signal that this production model of health care is widely accepted. It is clear that when nurses are asked to adopt this notion of outcomes, the practice of nursing is in danger of becoming routinized, with the one nursed

suffering the experience of objectification and depersonalization. A production model of outcomes of nursing care, coupled with a technologically dense environment, make it extremely difficult for nurses to engage
in caring relationships with patients.

The theory of Nursing As Caring (Boykin & Schoenhofer, 1993) provides a conceptual framework for integrating values, intentions, and expressions of nursing grounded in caring. Practice grounded in this
theoretical perspective is "not concerned with diagnosis of a problem to
be addressed through nursing but rather with participating in a mutual
relationship in which the nurse seeks to know the nursed in their unique,
unfolding expressions of caring" (Schoenhofer & Boykin, 1998, p. 10).
The unique role of the nurse in any health care situation, even those
laden with complex biomedical technologies, is to witness and nurture
the nursed as a person, as one who is living caring uniquely, moment
to moment, with aspirations of growing in caring ways. This way of
nursing occurs within the "nursing situation," a shared lived experience
in which the caring between the nurse and nursed enhances personhood
(Boykin & Schoenhofer, 1993, p. 33). The nurse participates in enhancing
personhood, a way of living grounded in caring, or as Mayeroff (1972)
has said, living the meaning of one's own life. As intentionally practiced,
Nursing As Caring assures that the patient is known and valued as person, and brings a needed emphasis to high-technology situations where
depersonalization is an ever-present possibility. Nursing use of any biomedical technology on behalf of the patient must be undertaken as an
avenue to knowing, acknowledging, affirming, and celebrating the patient as caring person. The artificial dichotomy between time to attend
to machines and time to care can be put to rest when nurses attend to
machines as an intentional expression of caring for person. In the practice
of Nursing As Caring, technological competence is not an end in itself
but an expression of intentional caring (Locsin, 1998).

From the perspective of Nursing As Caring, the concern of the health
care community with outcomes as economic and medical indicators is
expanded and personalized. The notion of outcomes of care is understood in a new way as the values experienced within the nursing situation (Boykin & Schoenhofer, 1997). It is not intended that this nursing
concept of outcomes replace the types of outcomes that are of interest to
medical and economic interests, but that it stand as an additional view
that nursing is accountable for representing. Documenting the personal
value experienced in a caring relationship re-personalizes the overall picture of what patients gain in their health care–seeking encounters.

Values experienced within the nursing situation, outcomes of caring
in nursing, cannot be predicted. Persons are not machines whose outputs
can be engineered. Human beings, including nurses and those they
nurse, are multidimensional. Persons live their human lives in the con-

text of complex and dynamic value systems—choosing, dreaming, creating. The following examples from real nursing situations suggest some possible "outcomes."

Vignette Number 1

Jason was a young man, a member of a cultural group in which manhood is a predominant feature of male identity. Jason was brought to the postsurgical recovery suite following a testicular biopsy. He was accompanied by the surgeon, who told Dan, the nurse, not to reveal the findings to Jason. Dan entered into an internal struggle with his nursing values, thinking, "I, nurse, must always and ever regard the person nursed from a position of love. I must enter all nursing activity with the sole purpose of using truth, only and ever, to promote the spiritual growth in the person nursed. In this climate of openness to myself and the other, we can begin to experience freedom from fear" (Boykin & Schoenhofer, 1993, p. 49). While Dan was struggling with his commitment to honesty as a way of caring, he removed Jason's endotracheal tube. Jason's eyes were filled with tears and he cried from the depths of his being, "I heard him. Why me, God?" (p. 49). In the 30 minutes that Dan remained with Jason, he made use of monitoring equipment, technologies of respiratory, hemodynamic, and neurological assessment, and all the other protective and supportive ways of caring for persons recovering from anesthesia following surgery. Dan did not carry out those procedures mechanically or thoughtlessly; they were part of his expression of caring and love for this person in this moment, Jason. In addition, Dan sat by Jason's side, held his hand, stroked his shoulder, encouraging Jason to rest, to trust in God to help him, to have strength, courage, and hope. What were the outcomes of post-anesthesia care? Observable, documentable outcomes in relation to the existing protocol were recorded: minimal bleeding, minimal discomfort, patient awake and responsive, vital signs within acceptable limits. These reported outcomes of Dan's care are important—and incomplete. They do not tell the whole story. Because of the short-term nature of the nursing relationship in a postanesthesia recovery setting, we cannot report with any certainty the values Jason experienced in the nursing situation. But was the relationship short-term? Dan says, "I will never forget Jason. He brought me closer to understanding honesty as caring" (Boykin & Schoenhofer, 1993, p. 50). We do not know if Dan's expression of caring kept their relationship alive in Jason's heart. Personal life experiences of mutual caring provide a knowledge base for suggesting possible values experienced by Jason in his nursing relationship with Dan. Jason may have experienced the value of human connectedness in a time of fear and despair, being sustained in his desire to trust and to hope. If we accept for a moment that

Jason would confirm this value experience, what might be the medical and economic implications? The personal implications? Sustained in trust and hope, Jason may decide to cooperate in medical treatment advice, and such cooperation ("compliance") would likely lead to the most cost-effective short- and long-term outcome. Over and above medical and economic outcomes of health care, Jason may find the hope and courage to modify his self-concept constructively, to enter into future caring relationships, to offer hope and courage to others in traumatic situations. If these outcomes were to occur, it cannot be said that they were created or produced through Dan's caring. It may be said, however, that Dan participated in Jason's enhanced personhood, his new ways of living his life as caring person.

Vignette Number 2

Changes in reimbursement structures have made home health nursing an increasingly technology-dense environment. What has not changed is the home health nurse's inclusion of family members as an important aspect of home nursing care. Patricia's assignment was to visit a person with AIDS in his home to monitor and support his use of intravenous pharmacotherapeutic technologies. Patricia observed as the patient's mother, Joyce, gave her son, Anthony, an injection and changed the injection site on his central venous catheter line. During the technological procedure, mother and son, with Patricia's supportive presence, engaged in a much-desired and long-deferred dialogue. Patricia noted, "The conversation was sparkling with humor and piercing with honesty, and created in my mind's eye a rich, colorful mosaic of years of love, beauty, and truth. Tonight I wish I were an artist so I could capture this vision on canvas" (Boykin & Schoenhofer, 1993, p. 54). When the procedure was completed, the moment of connectedness continued as all three gathered around the piano to sing family favorites.

Requests were offered by each member of the family, and within minutes Joyce was sitting next to me on the piano bench, singing loudly and punctuating words with feelings and strength and lending incredible meaning to the lyrics of "Old Man River." The deep, low, rumbling of the piano and purposefully driving tempo was responded to in kind with Joyce stamping her foot with each beat and pounding her knee with each word as she emphatically sang, "He just keeps rolling, he keeps on rolling along" (Boykin & Schoenhofer, 1993, p. 55).

As Patricia was going, Anthony said, "Thank you for helping my mother to smile" (p. 55). What outcomes would likely be recorded from this home nursing visit? What outcomes, values experienced in the nursing situation, would go unrecorded but for the courage of the nurse in languaging the beauty of the nursing situation in which personhood was clearly enhanced?

Vignette Number 3

Charles was a middle-aged man, husband and father of a young son, who had been on dialysis for 20 years. He came to a freestanding dialysis center several times a week, where he participated in a caring nursing relationship with Mark. Charles remarked on the sense of family connectedness among the clients and staff of the center. He described the experience of being cared for in the vigilance of the staff, their readiness to answer questions, and their welcoming inclusion of him as the active participant in his dialysis that he wanted to be. Charles said Mark and the other staff were "with him" in the way that he tried to be with his young son, as ready and caring teachers. Charles was training to be a dialysis counselor and said that the staff were his role models. Mark communicated deep respect for Charles as a person, and Charles's commitment to his own effective self-care strengthened Mark's resolve go the extra mile in his caregiving. Charles sought and received highly competent technological care from Mark and other staff members. He recounted a sudden and frightening episode of cardiac irregularity during dialysis, saying, "like a swarm of bees, there came the EKG machine and everything in the snap of a finger . . . it's that type of care, that knowing what to do, and all the time keeping me where I wasn't scared."

The "outcome" of that episode would typically be reported in terms of restoration to normal cardiac rhythm. That surely was one outcome of the caring Charles experienced in the nursing relationship; however, Charles himself provided a more holistic picture of the meaning and value of emergency technology used on his behalf. Much of the self-confidence with which Charles lived his relatively normal life, despite serious health challenges, was a reflection of the confidence, the faith, and trust he experienced in his nursing relationship with Mark. Charles trusted Mark completely to provide the knowledge and self-care skills he wanted in a way that had meaning for him. He experienced being known as a person in his own right, worthwhile, competent, a caring person. This knowing inspired Charles's desire to extend the hand of caring connectedness to others living with dialysis. The primary outcome of this technology-dependent nursing situation that is of interest to medicine and to those concerned with health care finance is that Charles was able to maintain a long-term positive health status that did not require hospitalization. Without discounting this outcome, it is clear that other outcomes, values experienced in the ongoing nursing situation, contributed significantly to the quality of life that Charles enjoyed. These quality-of-life outcomes played a significant role in Charles's decisions to decline home dialysis and to continue at the dialysis center, rather than transferring to one associated with his attending physician's practice. The values of "being with," respect, and participatory care contributed also to Charles's sense of himself as a competent father and contributing member of society. Without the language of nursing and the voice of nurses, these latter outcomes would remain largely unacknowledged, and treated as though they did not count.

CONCLUDING REMARKS

The deeply human outcomes suggested in these vignettes reflect the fundamental nature of nursing as a personal caring relationship. The most significant outcomes, those most meaningful to the persons involved in the caring relationships of nursing, are not amenable to accounting procedures. The meaning of nursing is lost in the impersonal, homogenized format of outcomes language—lost to those whose practices intersect that of nursing; to those who organize, manage, and finance health care systems; and to those who formulate health care policy. These vignettes demonstrate, however, that the meaning of nursing is not lost to nurses and those they nurse. Nurses who practice in high-technology settings and patients who seek care in those environments continue to experience the value of caring in nursing. No practice settings are in greater need of the humanizing care of nursing than technology-dense environments. To assure that the caring that is nursing is fully acknowledged and valued, nurses must create effective forms of communicating "outcomes" of their practice. Nurses must speak, and speak in the language of nursing—the language of caring—so that the value of nursing is recognized and supported. Nurses who practice from the framework of Nursing As Caring find courageous and innovative ways of speaking: recording the fullness of their care in the patient chart; portraying nursing in aesthetic modes such as poetry; telling stories of nursing in the board room as well as in the break room.

REFERENCES

Boykin, A., & Schoenhofer, S. (1993). *Nursing as caring: A model for transforming practice*. New York: National League for Nursing.

Boykin, A., & Schoenhofer, S. (1997). Reframing outcomes: Enhancing personhood. *Advanced Practice Nursing Quarterly, 3*, 60–65.

Fess, P. E., Warren, C. S., & Reeve, J. M. (Eds.). (1993). *Accounting Principles* (17th ed.). Cincinnati: South-Western.

Locsin, R. C. (1998). Technologic competence as caring in critical care nursing. *Holistic Nursing Practice, 12*(4), 50–56.

Mayeroff, M. (1972). *On caring.* New York: HarperPerennial.

Schoenhofer, S. O., & Boykin, A. (1998). The value of caring experienced in nursing. *International Journal for Human Caring, 2*(3), 9–15.

Chapter 8

Practicing Nursing: Technological Competency as an Expression of Caring

Rozzano C. Locsin

Her name is Flo and she is a nurse unlike any you have ever met. She can perform "nurse" duties. Remind you to take your medicine. Take your vital signs and even e-mail them to your doctor. If she does a good job, though, don't bother patting her on the back, because Flo doesn't respond to such positive reinforcement. She is a robot, a robo nurse. (Gutierrez, 2000)

The traditional question "what is nursing?" continues to be asked, reflecting the growth of nursing as a discipline of knowledge and a practice profession. Its seeming constancy as a question is often ascribed to the perennial use of the word "nurse" referring to the performance of tasks, and as a consequence of the persisting image of nursing practice as tasks. The creation of the "robo nurse," a complex piece of machinery that, in human fashion, is made to perform technical "nurse" activities such as taking a person's temperature, perpetuates this image. The "nurse," a robot, simply facilitates completion of tasks for people. The persistent image of nursing as accomplishing tasks undeniably makes "Flo" a nurse.

The purpose of this chapter is to describe practicing nursing as technological competency—an expression of caring in nursing. The advent of medical technology, and its domination as the major influence in health care, places nursing in the awkward position of being dependent upon competencies for these technologies in order to engage in practice. Practicing nursing as caring through technological competency is the achievement of knowing persons in their wholeness by the authentic, intentional, knowledgeable, and efficient use of technologies of nursing. These technologies influence the appreciation of nursing as integral to persons' well-being, allowing the nurse to participate in the process of knowing persons in their wholeness. The ultimate purpose of technological competency is to acknowledge persons in their wholeness. Such acknowledgment compels the redesigning of processes of nursing—ways of expressing, celebrating, and appreciating the practice of nursing as knowing persons.

Patients need to know what is occurring in their care. In a recent study by Hupcey and Zimmerman (2000), it was found that "Critically ill patients have a strong need to know throughout and after their time in the intensive care unit" (p. 192). This finding suggests that nurses participate in revealing ways that answer to the clients' need to know about what they have undergone in the intensive care unit, and what will happen to them in the future. Practicing nursing in order to know persons in their wholeness epitomizes this participation. The nurse facilitates the design, development, and implementation of ways of nursing, enhancing participation of patients so that they can better celebrate the experience of being a patient. Nurturing persons in their wholeness grounded in caring (Boykin & Schoenhofer, 1993) exemplifies this process of nursing. Using technologies of nursing in purposeful ways in order to know persons in their wholeness makes nursing practice more meaningful.

Nursing As Caring (Boykin & Schoenhofer, 1993) grounds the practice of technological competency in nursing. From a practice perspective, technological competency is proficiency in devices such as machines, instruments, and tools, and a manifestation of being caring in nursing. Essentially, technological competency as an expression of caring in nursing is the relevant use of these technologies for the ultimate purpose of knowing persons in their wholeness. In this practice of nursing, technology is used not to know "what is the person?" but rather, to know "who is the person?"

DESCRIPTION OF NURSING PRACTICE

Gadamer (1991) explains that "practice is a communally developed way of being that promotes human good. A practice is concerned not only with how to bring about the good, but what good or value is worth pursuing" (p. 83). The ANA Code for Nurses (1985), describes nursing practice as focusing on the achievement of health promotion and illness prevention. While this may be the ideal, nursing practitioners in their preferred practice arenas are not provided with many such opportunities. Contemporary practice settings often preferred by nursing practitioners are intensive and critical care units where the desired qualification is technological proficiency. The advent of machine technologies, which perform medical tasks of determining the functional status of human organs and systems, has created an alternative practice focus for nurses in these technologically dependent care settings. While it is necessary to understand the operation of machine devices for the purpose of understanding the functioning human being, their use ought not to consign persons to being regarded as objects. The objectification of persons becomes an ordinary occurrence in situations where the practice of nursing is merely understood as achievement of tasks.

TECHNOLOGICAL COMPETENCY AS AN EXPRESSION OF CARING IN NURSING

To professional nurses, activities involving machine technologies, such as monitoring ventilators and electrocardiograms (EKGs), create overwhelming demands on being technologically competent. Activities such as interpreting data from cardiac monitors, manipulating ventilators and intravenous pumps, or even the skill of starting intravenous lines are frequently recognized as demonstrations of technological competency, rather than as expressions of caring in nursing. In situations where technologies are used to know "what" is the patient rather than "who" is the patient, the authentic intention to know persons in their wholeness is often devalued (Locsin, 1998).

The practice of nursing in critical care settings is typified by expressions of technological competency. Grounding such a practice on the perspective of Nursing As Caring (Boykin & Schoenhofer, 1993) allows for the celebration of persons in their wholeness. Because the practice is nursing, exhibiting technological competency as caring in nursing simultaneously reveals the harmonious coexistence between technology and caring (Locsin, 1995). In today's health care structure, the major characteristic desired of health care personnel is technological proficiency. Patient satisfaction usually focuses on how well their recovery was facilitated by the nurse, which, for the most part is associated with competency in using machine technologies (Locsin, 1998).

Often, nursing practitioners declare that the demands of technological competency in technology-dependent settings are so arduous that true caring is no longer possible. In this association, "caring" usually means activities performed with the patient, such as holding the patient's hand or being physically present and interacting. These activities are empirical examples of the nature of being with the patient from the traditional view of a caring nurse. While being with the patient may be an expression of a "feeling, caring nurse," many perceive this caring nursing practice as time spent or wasted, and actions undertaken that do not influence the health of patients, and which therefore, are expendable. To some nurses, activities that are technology-based often seem uncaring, but to technologically competent nurses, these are normal activities reflecting nursing in critical care settings (Locsin, 1998).

TECHNOLOGIES IN NURSING

Technology is described as a means to an end, an instrument, and a human activity (Heidegger, 1977), and is traditionally viewed as equipment and techniques. Technology comprises methods and expressions that delineate structures and procedures in techniques. Technique however, is a standard procedure that can be taught, a recipe that can be duplicated, and that, when followed, always leads to the desired end. Fetal monitoring, in vitro fertilization, and artificial insemination are easily identified as techniques that are aspects of reproduction technology (Zwolski, 1989). In nursing, technology is expressed in procedures and techniques that facilitate nursing activities. Technique is exemplified by the "nursing process," a recipe that, when followed, illustrates the mechanistic view of nursing practice.

The level of knowledge the nurse possesses is not what makes the person the focus of nursing. Instead, it is the intentional and authentic presence (Paterson & Zderad, 1988) brought into the situation that enables the nurse to know the other as a person living unique hopes, dreams, and aspirations. Nursing technologies that are enacted for the sole purpose of procedural efficiency only sustain the impression that nursing practice is simply technological competency (Locsin, 1998).

Competency is recognized and advocated as an effective component of technology in nursing practice (Girot, 1993; Miller et al., 1993). The rapid development of technology and its increased utility in health care have contributed to this phenomenon. Miller et al. (1993) ascribe two meanings to competence: (1) competence equated with performance and referred to descriptively as an activity, and (2) competence as a quality or state of being of an individual. In the former meaning, competence is easily envisioned as the product, while the latter meaning exhibits a characteristic of one who performs the activity. These attributes highlight the description of competency as meaningful and distinctive to the practice of nursing (Miller et al., 1993). Expert nurses use these meanings intuitively in providing care and in using theory in their practice (Benner, 1984).

PRACTICING NURSING AS TECHNOLOGICAL COMPETENCY

The pressure to achieve technological proficiency in nursing practice has inspired re-visioning of the technology–caring dichotomy (Locsin, 1995). Beginning in the 1970s, with the nursing dialogue centered on care versus cure, research in nursing has since focused on nursing knowledge development, with nursing practice as the focal arena. The prominence that caring has gained as a central expression of nursing is evidence of this emphasis. Current importance ascribed to technology is a signal of the successful incorporation of technological competency as caring in nursing. Levine (1995) asserts:

There is much theorizing left to do and practitioners are needed to help identify it. . . . Technology is not going to go away and nurses need to deal with it—not as technical automatons, but as expert scientists skilled in the interpretation and use of the technology of health care. Why not a theory of nursing that properly integrates the human person and the technology needed in patient care? What about theories that will help nurses care for the increased severity of the hospitalized sick? (pp. 13–14)

Technology has the potential to bring the patient closer to the nurse by enhancing the nurse's ability to know more about the person. Conversely, technology can also increase the gap between the nurse and client, as exhibited by the conscious disregard of the patient as person, and ignorance of the nursing imperative to know the patient as person. Technology defines a familiar work world for the critical care nurse, but it also can contribute to the alienation of the patient (Porter, 1992).

EXPRESSING TECHNOLOGICAL COMPETENCY AS CARING

Concepts implicit in the theory of Nursing As Caring (Boykin & Schoenhofer, 1993) ground technological competency as caring in nursing—a way in which technology and caring are unified in the practice of nursing. A nurse who is technologically proficient but does not know the patient fully as a person in the moment is the ultimate example of one who is simply a technologist. Understanding technological competency as having humanistic implications and meaning, and realizing that caring in various settings is expressed through all nursing activities, even those that are technological activities, makes this harmonious unification possible (Locsin, 1998).

Persons grow in their competency to express themselves as caring persons (Boykin & Schoenhofer, 1993). This competency may well be conceived as the nurse's caring demonstrated as technological competency while being authentically present with the patient. To appreciate technological competency as caring, its use as a means to an end and as a human activity must reflect intention-to-nurse (Purnell & Locsin, 2000), and technological responsibility. It is in this context that the nurse is challenged to care (Cooper, 1993).

Nurses who respond to patients' specific calls for nursing portray technological competency as an expression of caring in nursing. These calls for nursing may be from health conditions that are monitored by multiple pieces of technical equipment such as ventilators, cardiac monitors, multiple intravenous lines, and blood gas monitoring requirements. The nurse is challenged to be technologically proficient while responding authentically and intentionally to calls for nursing. Such authenticity and intentionality is demonstrated when the nurse, with all the demands of technological expertise, accepts the patient fully as a human being, not as an object.

Jones and Alexander (1993) proclaimed that "the adoption of a nontraditional nursing definition of technology, which incorporates caring, will contribute to the growth and evolution of nursing" (p. 19). The nurse uses technology to know the person, one who is in the process of living and growing in caring.

THE PROCESS OF NURSING IN A TECHNOLOGICALLY DENSE ENVIRONMENT

Technological competency as caring in nursing involves intentionality with compassion, confidence, commitment, and conscience as requisites to caring in nursing (Phillips, 1993). This is where the process of nursing takes on a focus different from the traditional series of problem-solving actions. By donning the lens of Nursing As Caring (Boykin & Schoenhofer, 1993), technological competency as caring in nursing can be acknowledged. With such visionary lenses, nursing is expressed as the simultaneous, momentary interconnectedness between the nurse and the patient. The nurse relies on the patient for "calls for nursing." These calls are specific mechanisms which patients use, and provide the opportunity for the nurse to respond with the authentic intention of knowing the other fully as a caring person. Calls for nursing may be expressed as hopes and desires, such as hoping to be free from pain or from complications of disease and treatments, or simply the desperate desire to go home, or to die peacefully. As uniquely as these nursing situations are expressed, the critical care nurse is challenged to "hear" these calls for nursing, and to respond authentically and intentionally in nurturing persons. These appropriate nursing responses may be communicated as patterns of relating information, such as those derived from machines like the EKG monitor in order to know the physiological status of the patient, or to administer lifesaving medications, institute transfer plans, or to refer patients to other health care professionals.

The challenge of nursing is expressing technological competency as caring, ably focusing on the other as caring person, whole and complete in the moment and growing in caring from moment to moment. Every human being uniquely responds to personal conditions in the moment. The nurse understands that the process of nursing occurs without preconceived views that categorize persons as needing to be "fixed," like fitting individuals into a "box" of predicted conditions. By allowing the patient to unfold as a person and to live fully as a human being, the nurse facilitates the goal of nursing in the "caring between," enhancing personhood (Boykin & Schoenhofer, 1993).

Nursing practitioners long for a practice of nursing that is based on the authentic desire to know patients fully as human beings rather than as objects. Through this authentic intention and desire, nurses are challenged to use every creative, imaginative, and innovative way possible to appreciate and celebrate the patient's intentions to live fully and grow as a human being. Only with expertise in technologies of nursing can technological competence as an expression of caring in nursing be realized.

Technological competency demonstrated from a perspective not grounded in nursing is the ultimate impersonation of a nurse: simply being technologically competent is not nursing (Locsin, 1998). Nursing occurs in situations when technologies are exercised proficiently with the authentic intention to know patients fully as persons who are in the process of living and growing in caring (Boykin & Schoenhofer, 1993). When viewed from this nursing perspective, technological competency as an expression of caring is truly nursing.

Nursing practitioners must find meaning in their nursing and express this meaning in ways that are clearly recognizable as nursing practice, rather than as medical practice or even technical practice. Describing nursing practice as completion of tasks does not serve the profession well. Nurses are urged to value technological competency as an expression of caring in nursing and integral to health care. Otherwise, the image of the robot nurse, simply facilitating completion of tasks for people, undeniably makes "Flo" a nurse.

REFERENCES

American Nurses Association (ANA). (1985). Code for nurses. Washington, DC: ANA.

Benner, P. (1984). From novice to expert. Menlo Park, CA: Addison-Wesley.

Bishop, A., & Scudder, J. (1997). Nursing as a practice rather than an art or a science. Nursing Outlook, 45(2), 82–85.

Boykin, A., & Schoenhofer, S. (1993). Nursing as caring: A model for transforming practice. New York: National League for Nursing Press.

Cooper, M. (1993). The intersection of technology and care in the ICU. Advances in Nursing Science, 15(3), 23–32.

Gadamer, H., & Lawrence, F. (Trans.). (1991). Reason in the age of innocence. Cambridge, MA: MIT Press.

Girot, E. (1993). Assessment of competence in clinical practice: A phenomeno-logical approach. *Journal of Advanced Nursing, 8*, 114–119.

Gutierrez, L. (2000, March 1). Robo nurse? *Palm Beach Post*, 3D.

Heidegger, M. (1977). *The question concerning technology and other essays*. New York: Harper and Row.

Hupcey, J., & Zimmerman, H. (2000). The need to know: Experiences of critically ill patients. *American Journal of Critical Care, 9*(3), 192–198.

Jones, C., & Alexander, J. (1993). The technology of caring: A synthesis of tech-nology and caring for nursing administration. *Nursing Administration Quarterly, 17*(2), 11–20.

Leininger, M. (1988). Leininger's theory of nursing: Cultural care diversity and universality. *Nursing Science Quarterly, 1*, 152–160.

Levine, M. (1995). The rhetoric of nursing theory. *Image: Journal of Nursing Schol-arship, 27*(1), 13–14.

Locsin, R. (1995). Machine technologies and caring in nursing. *Image: Journal of Nursing Scholarship, 27*(3), 201–203.

Locsin, R. (1997). Knowing the whole person: Revolutionizing nursing practice. *The University of Iceland, Nursing Research Paper Series, 1* (suppl.), 359–362.

Locsin, R. (1998). Technological competency as caring in critical care nursing. *Holistic Nursing Practice, 12*(4), 50–56.

Miller, C., Hoggan, J., Pringle, S., & West, G. (1993). Credit where credit is due. The report of the accreditation of work-based learning project 1988. In E. Girot, Assessment of competence in clinical practice: A phenomenological approach. *Journal of Advanced Nursing, 8*, 114–119.

Paterson, J., & Zderad, P. (1988). *Humanistic nursing*. New York: National League for Nursing.

Phillips, P. (1993). A deconstruction of caring. *Journal of Advanced Nursing, 18*, 1554–1558.

Porter, S. (1992). The poverty of professionalization: A critical analysis of strat-egies for the occupational advancement of nursing. *Journal of Advanced Nursing, 17*, 723–728.

Purnell, M., & Locsin, R. (2000). *Intentionality: Unification in nursing*. Manuscript submitted for publication.

Roach, S. (1987). *The human act of caring*. Ottawa: Canadian Hospital Association.

Watson, J. (1985). *Nursing: The philosophy and science of caring*. Boulder: Colorado Associated University Press.

Zwolski, K. (1989). Professional nursing in a technical system. *Image: Journal of Nursing Scholarship, 21*(4), 238–242.

Chapter 9

On the Relationship between Technique and Dehumanization

Alan Barnard

INTRODUCTION

Technology has evolved from being a component of life that reflected the cultural, spiritual, and contextual nuances of unique communities and groups to being a phenomenon that transforms society and the workplace. It transforms what nurses do and how nursing practice is organized and conceived, and the values nurses espouse. Nurses have identified some of these transformations, and nursing literature contains ongoing debate on its benefits and costs. Technology has been described as advancing the profession, care delivery, roles and responsibilities, skills, knowledge, and nursing management (Gordon, 1992; Leach, 1990; Simpson & Brown, 1985). Alternative description has emphasized a lack of caring and an inability of nurses to provide emotional support for patients that is more than reassurance about machinery, procedures, and policies (Calne, 1994; Hawthorne & Yurkovich, 1995). The debate reflects concepts and issues that have been considered in philosophy of technology literature over the past 200 years. Philosophy of technology develops when a person or group make technology the foreground or central focus of reflection, scholarship, and research. Two differing foci of reflection have been identified, and are described as engineering and humanities philosophy of technology. Engineering philosophy of technology examines the nature of technology in terms of technical use. Emphasis is placed on its concepts, methods, design, and objective presence. Humanities philosophy of technology accepts the engineering focus, but expands on it to include not only the object or agent of use, but also human experience, society, and culture. Technology is examined in relation to, for example, religion, poetry, politics, and gender (Barnard, 2000c; Mitcham, 1994). Although philosophy of technology has not been identified as a specific area of reflection within nursing knowledge, the dominant focus of attention in nursing has been from an engineering perspective, even though in recent years increasing consideration is being given to gender, caring, and politics (Barnard, 1997; Fairman & D'Antonio, 1999; Rudge, 1999; Sandelowski, 1999). Two of many questions about technology that remain unanswered within nursing relate to whether it influences caring and causes the dehumanization of people and groups. For example, it has been claimed that technology is associated with alienation, dehumanization, and a deterioration of nursing practice, values, goals, and ideals (Allan & Hall, 1988; Calne, 1994; Cooper, 1993; Donley, 1991).

This chapter examines dehumanization within the context of technology and nursing. Its thesis is that dehumanization can and does occur in association with technology, but is less attributable to specific types of technology, such as machinery, equipment, chemicals, utensils, automata, tools, clothes, and utilities (technical objects), than it is to the influence of a technological system referred to often as technique. Although technique can refer to behaviors and activities associated with performing an action or procedure, in this instance it refers to the development of rational and efficient human, economic, political, and organizational systems used for the advancement of technology as an integral part of modern health care and nursing. Discussion begins with an examination of the meanings of both technology and dehumanization, and is followed by exploration of the concept of technique within the context of contemporary nursing practice.

WHAT IS TECHNOLOGY?

Technology is a complex interrelationship between numerous influential characteristics that include technical objects, people, organizations, science, culture, gender, society, values, and politics, based on the goals of efficiency and logical order. Technology is the manifestation of our desire to make and use tools in the world around us. At its most obvious, technology refers to current, antiquated, and failed technical objects that are developed for use and application in nursing, health care, and society.

However, technology is manifest also as knowledge and skills associated with the various types of technology that nurses use, repair (e.g., troubleshoot), design, and assess on a daily and ongoing basis in the various domains of practice. In addition, it manifests itself as the ways nursing practice is organized into a system (technique). The act of including technical objects in nursing introduces patterns of technological activity that by their very nature influence the way nurses organize the profession, patient care, knowledge, skills, roles, and responsibilities. Failure to identify and acknowledge all the various ways technology manifests itself leads to inadequate interpretation of technology within the contexts of nursing (Barnard, 1996, 1999; Ellul, 1964, 1980; Fairman, 1996; Fairman & D'Antonio, 1999; Feenberg, 1999; Winner, 1977).

THE MEANING OF DEHUMANIZATION

Dehumanization refers to the loss of identity and community through objectification or denial of human attributes associated with self, body, and personality, and is an experience associated with technology (Calne, 1994; Cooper, 1993; Mann, 1992). It involves the negation of social and cultural origins, an objectification of the personal, and a rejection of those specific attributes that make each person who they are at any one time. It is characterized by the deprivation of qualities associated with meaning, interest, and compassion. When dehumanization occurs, there is a loss of humanness and the fostering of a perception that individuals and groups are understood best in terms of biology, disease, machinery, or animals (Harvey, 1985; Kelman, 1973). For example, the value of an individual is lost when he or she is identified or labeled in accordance with a disease or treatment (i.e., the cholecystectomy in bed 7 or the catheter in bed 8). Dehumanization has been linked to clinical environments in which patients have little influence over decision making, have limited choice in relation to care, and experience health care surrounded by equipment, noise, and activity (e.g., an intensive care unit or a complex and busy surgical or medical ward) (Green, 1992; Merideth & Edworthy, 1995).

Dehumanization is different from depersonalization because the latter is related to experiences of unreality involving the self and the external world, and feelings of being split or cut off from one's body. However, accepted features of depersonalization are confounded by factors such as the lack of an agreed ordinary or common state of consciousness, the influence of past experience, emotional maturity, how an individual reacts to external trauma, and its manifestation as a defense mechanism to protect an individual through denial of factors external to the body (e.g., "this is not happening to me") (Levy & Wachtel, 1979).

Nonetheless, despite the fact that experiences associated with both dehumanization and depersonalization can and do occur, the term "dehumanization" is unhelpful when thinking about technology. For example, the term has been associated with deterministic inclinations to blame machinery and automata for uncaring experiences, and explanation of what is truly human does not often accompany accusations of dehumanization. In answer to this dilemma, Winner (1977) suggests that a better approach to expressing the relationship between technology and dehumanization is that "more highly developed, rational-artificial structures tend to overwhelm and replace less well developed forms of life. That is, the organized and efficient world of technology has a tendency to dominate over the less conscious and spontaneous world of patients and nursing practice. Organized and efficient contemporary health care practices can influence negatively the expression of caring, the judicious use of technical objects, the practice of nursing, and the experience of patients" (p. 212).

TECHNIQUE AND NURSING

With modern nursing that is technologically dependent, with machinery and automata increasingly influencing our lives, it is important to focus not only on technical objects as the reason to label modern nursing or contemporary health care as technological. Emphasizing technical objects identifies that which is impressive and obvious about technological society, but inadequately informs us of what is unique about modern times.

Technology has, to a greater or lesser extent, always been part of nursing. The use of technical objects at this time, even though they are increasingly more advanced and sophisticated, does not constitute a criterion for defining contemporary nursing practice as technological. Nurses have always used tools, chemicals, potions, equipment, and so on, to manipulate and interact with people, disease, and the world around them. If the development of technology in the form of technical objects is the reason for referring to contemporary nursing and society as technological, then all nursing practices and societies (past, present, and future) must be included under the term (Barnard, 1996; Ellul, 1964; Purcell, 1994; Winner, 1977).

However, the term "technological society" is a common idiom for Western society. It originates from authors such as Ellul (1964), who argued that since the industrial revolution a new relationship has emerged between technology and society, based on the establishment of technique. That is, the formation of a system or order aimed at the absolute efficiency of methods and means (for a given stage of development) in every field of human endeavor. His aim was to highlight the features of modern technology and explain their significance to contemporary society. Ellul's sociological/philosophical arguments were concerned with the relationship between technology and politics, economics, people, and theology, rather than specific pessimism about the use of technical objects, although he does predict technique will increasingly control our lives. His analysis is at times fatalistic, however, and does not acknowledge adequately the importance of social construction in the development of technology. For example, technical designs are based not only on technique, but also on sociocultural meanings that are gendered and incorporate assumptions related to nursing, health care, society, values, and dominant interests. Notwithstanding, technique remains a major component of modern technology, and nurses need to confront it in practice and theory. Sociocultural meanings, politics, and the fostering of an efficient and rational order (technique) are equally backgrounds or external horizons that constitute hermeneutic dimensions of technology (Barnard, 1996, 1998, 2000b; Ellul, 1964; Feenberg, 1999; Mitcham, 1994).

FROM NATURAL TO ARTIFICIAL

Science has revealed many structures, processes, and laws of nature, and provided nursing with knowledge previously known only to God. Knowledge and understanding have expanded and many societies have experienced direct benefit. However, from the perspective of technology a second event has been occurring, not only in nursing and health care, but globally. Through the emergence of technique, many aspects of the natural milieu have been rationalized, arranged, and standardized in the search for greater efficiency. A technical order is being created that proliferates a new relationship with technology, based on seven features that are described as rationality, artificiality, technical automation, self-augmentation, monism, universalism, and autonomy (Ellul, 1964, 1980).

The importance of acknowledging technique as a characteristic of technology continues to be emphasized in many philosophies of technology (Janicaud, 1994; Mitcham, 1994). For example, Feenberg (1999) argues that technique is the foundation of a secondary instrumentalization that is described as systemization, mediation, vocation, and initiative. It is argued that in technological society, technique is integrated with the natural to bring about technical and social environments that support the instrumental functions of technology.

In modern nursing and society, technique structures collective behavior increasingly, and influences individual lives and professional perspectives. Tradition is replaced by discovery, using and consuming replaces making and using, and nature is replaced by a system of arrangements and control. Many aspects of nursing become ordered in accordance with technical demands, not in any abstract, planned, or theoretical manner, but as a result of interrelationships that develop between multiple subsystems. This is the reason why contemporary nursing can be described as technological. Technique opposes the incorporation of subjective and non-technical phenomenon by enframing them into the rational and organized order of technology. According to Mitcham (1994), its challenge is that it "resists incorporation into or subordination to non-technical attitudes and ways of thinking. It explains other actions as forms of itself and thereby transforms them into itself. It constitutes, as it were, the social manifestation of Heidegger's Ge-stell" (p. 59).

Technique influences nursing through education, economics, media, organizational structures, politics, and people. It can assist nurses by providing stability when, for example, there is a lack of supervision in nursing practice, such as the availability of a policy and procedure manual. Resources, facts, values, and people become ordered within efficient and effective, systematic arrangements that are sometimes to our benefit.

However, technique also determines causal processes and the primacy of means over ends, the reduction of individual differences, the maximization of efficiency, specialization of practice, the development of universal conformity, and an increasing sameness to product, processes, and thought (Ellul, 1964, 1980; Winner, 1977). Examples of technique in health care include economic rationalism, efficiency drives, diagnostic related groups, time and motion studies, and best practice models. Differences between tradition, culture, symbolism, artistic expression, and behaviors are reduced to demonstrable schemata, policies, organizational management, and educational goals. Notwithstanding, it should be noted that many participants in the process obtain exactly what they desire. The participating nurse obtains the pleasure of being part of a technological system, reassured by the predictable nature of its organization and efficiency. The patient obtains a sense of being part of technological health care that is manifest as control and predictable outcomes. However, if participation is not desired or appropriate, there can be feelings that nursing care has become standardized, the human condition has become subject to measurement, and the subjective and personal experiences of patients are secondary to technique (Allan, 1988; Barnard, 1997; Braun et al., 1984; Cooper, 1993; Henderson, 1980; Reiser, 1978).

TECHNIQUE, DEHUMANIZATION, AND IDEOLOGY: A DEFENSE OF THE NURSE

Some nurses have argued that through appropriate education, experience, insight, and a commitment to practice nursing as it ought to be practiced, nurses gain the potential and ability to focus on people rather than technology (Braun et al., 1984; Clifford, 1986; Raatikainen, 1989). Arguments have been based primarily on the primacy of professional values. Claims of success are unsubstantiated, however, and focus excessively on inexperience and the lack of appropriate education, skills, and commitment to explain dehumanization and alterations to caring. They are unreasonable at times, and reflect ideological contentions that do not acknowledge appropriately the challenges of modern technology.

For example, nurses are disenfranchised often within clinical environments. It is not always the case that nurses control technological processes along the entire length of their conception, nor their operation and outcome (means–end spectrum). Although experience, education, and commitment will encourage excellence in nursing practice, it is unclear whether nurses are capable always of achieving the professional values espoused.

Technology is not a neutral phenomenon and the effects of technique are predictable. For example, Barnard (1998) illustrated that the demands of technology can alter the will (volition) of surgical nurses (Barnard, 2000a; Barnard & Gerber, 1999). Technology can, to a greater or lesser extent, influence a nurse's capacity to accomplish practice goals, display caring behaviors, and maintain principles of practice, particularly when clinical practice is significant for its excessive policies, work overload, technical objects, protocols, and limited resources. The demands of checking equipment, enacting policies and procedures, responding to bureaucratic demands, administering drugs, answering telephones and responding to alarms, and so on, can be a compelling influence on a nurse's time, physical commitment, and intellectual attention. A tension is experienced sometimes between the control obtained through technology and the non-technical practice of nurses. The tension can create nursing practice that is understood to be increasingly frustrating and less responsive to the needs of individual patients. The ability of nurses to express many of the caring behaviors associated commonly with nursing (e.g., compassion) can be challenged, not by a lack of interest, experience, education, ability, or desire to be involved more with people, but by the influence of technology on the nurses' roles and responsibilities. Technology can modify a caring nurse's ability to express her or his concern for patients, despite a desire and commitment to do so. Efficiency, speed, precision, productivity, resource management, and technological progress become ends in themselves. Both the patient and nurse are subject potentially to experiences of dehumanization. Technique emphasizes the structural (what) of technical objects, and de-emphasizes the subjective-humanness of living. Under these conditions nursing practice that is authentic to the goals and intentions of practitioners is increasingly difficult. Nurses find it hard to act out ethical and moral ideals and to express humanistic and interpersonal qualities that are co-created and expressed at the time(s) when the nurse seeks to engage in a humanizing and caring moment.

CONCLUDING STATEMENTS

Technology is a major contributor in changing the way we live our lives, the practice of nursing, and the experience of health care. Technology is transformative and places demands on each nurse that are more than, but include, its instrumental application. Modern technology is responsible for increasingly shorter stays in hospitals, alteration to staffing, standardization, time constraints, and social, political, administrative, and economic arrangements. These consequences, combined with dominant social interests, increasing legal liability, and the maintenance of technical objects, produce nursing practices that are focused sometimes on functionality, sameness, conformity, automation, safety, efficiency, and logical order. The rational and efficient world of health care has a tendency to overwhelm the human and subjective world of patients and nurses. Therefore, excellence in nursing practice demands further involvement with issues related to ethical, gender, economic, theoretical, political, and intellectual aspects of technology (Allan, 1988; Barnard, 1997, 2000a, 2000c; Fairman, 1996; Harding, 1980; Rudge, 1999; Sandelowski, 1988, 1997).

Fundamental to diminishing dehumanization is the appropriate use of technology and examination of technique within the contexts of contemporary nursing practice. A beginning point to the process will be an ethic of non-power in which, at certain times and under certain conditions, the use of technology is resisted (Ellul, 1989). That is, for example, when the needs of patients do not warrant its use; when the expertise and time of nurses do not equate with the demands of machinery and automata; when the use of technology brings the imposition of unwanted professional, economic, political, and human efficiencies; and when humanization of care is increasingly less likely.

The growth of scientific and technological knowledge has produced enormous advances for nursing and health care. Technology assists nurses in many ways and the continued involvement of nursing with technology is appropriate, important, and exciting. Therefore, approaches to nursing practice are required that maximize the involvement of nurses with technology, and at the same time encourage responsiveness to the specifics of human experience. The advantages of modern technology need to be balanced against an ongoing struggle for a humane and caring world. The challenge for nursing is that, even though acceptance of all that technology brings to nursing and patient care is not always compulsory, selected rejection of technology and a renewed focus on humanizing care can (could) place nurses in an inferior position. Non-conformity to technique makes nursing unresponsive to the predominant agenda of technological health care (society). Productive critique that seeks ways for nurses to respond appropriately to technique is necessary, and will be an important future development for nursing practice and theory.

REFERENCES

Allan, J. D., & Hall, B. A. (1988). Challenging the focus on technology: A critique of the medical model in a changing health care system. *Advances in Nursing Science, 10*(3), 22–34.

Barnard, A. (1996). Technology and nursing: An anatomy of definition. *International Journal of Nursing Studies, 33*(4), 433–441.

Barnard, A. (1997). A critical review of the belief that technology is a neutral object and nurses are its master. *Journal of Advanced Nursing, 26*(1), 126–131.

Barnard, A. (1998). *Understanding technology in contemporary surgical nursing: A phenomenographic examination*. Unpublished Ph.D. diss., University of New England, Armidale, Australia.

Barnard, A. (1999). Technology and the Australian nursing experience. In J. Daly, S. Speedy, & D. Jackson (Eds.), *Contexts of nursing: An introduction* (pp. 163–176). Sydney: Maclennan & Petty.

Barnard, A. (2000a). Alteration to will as an experience of technology and nursing. *Journal of Advanced Nursing, 31*(5), 1136–1144.

Barnard, A. (2000b). Nursing technology as object: An examination. *Canadian Journal of Nursing Research* (in press).

Barnard, A. (2000c). Towards an understanding of technology and nursing practice. In J. Greenwood (Ed.), *Nursing theory in Australia: Development and application* (2nd ed.) (in press). Sydney: HarperCollins.

Barnard, A., & Gerber, R. (1999). Understanding technology in contemporary surgical nursing: A phenomenographic examination. *Nursing Inquiry, 6*(3), 157–170.

Braun, J. L., Baines, S. L., Olson, N. G., Scruby, L. S., Manteuffel, C. A., & Cretilli, P. K. (1984). The future of nursing: Combining humanistic and technological values. *Health Values: Achieving High Level Wellness, 8*(3), 12–15.

Calne, S. (1994). Dehumanization in intensive care. *Nursing Times, 90*(17), 31–33.

Clifford, C. (1986). Patients, relatives and nurses in a technological environment. *Intensive Care Nursing, 2*, 67–72.

Cooper, M. C. (1993). The intersection of technology and care in the ICU. *Advances in Nursing Science, 15*(3), 23–32.

Donley, R. (1991). Spiritual dimensions of health care: Nursing mission. *Nursing & Health Care, 12*(4), 178–183.

Ellul, J. (1964). *The technological society*. New York: Alfred A. Knopf.

Ellul, J. (1980). *The technological system*. New York: Continuum.

Ellul, J. (1989). The search for ethics in a technicist society. *Research in Philosophy and Technology, 9*, 23–36.

Fairman, J. (1996). Response to tools of the trade: Analyzing technology as object in nursing. *Scholarly Inquiry for Nursing Practice: An International Journal, 10*(1), 17–21.

Fairman, J., & D'Antonio, P. (1999). Virtual power: Gendering the nurse-technology relationship. *Nursing Inquiry, 6*, 178–186.

Feenberg, A. (1999). *Questioning technology*. New York: Routledge.

Gordon, S. (1992). The importance of being nurses. *Technology Review, 95*(7), 42–51.

Green, A. (1992). How nurses can ensure the sounds patients hear have a positive rather than negative effect upon recovery and quality of care. *Intensive and Critical Care, 8,* 245–248.

Harding, S. (1980). Value laden technologies and the politics of nursing. In S. F. Spicker & S. Gadow (Eds.), *Nursing: Images and ideals* (pp. 49–75). New York: Springer.

Harvey, J. (1985). Living between life and death. *New Society, 74*(1192), 233–236.

Hawthorne, D. L., & Yurkovich, N. J. (1995). Science, technology, caring and the professions: Are they compatible? *Journal of Advanced Nursing, 21*(6), 1087–1091.

Henderson, V. (1980). Preserving the essence of nursing in a technological age. *Journal of Advanced Nursing, 5*(3), 245–260.

Janicaud, D. (1994). *Powers of the rational: Science, technology, and the future of thought* (P. Birmingham & E. Birmingham, Trans.). Bloomington: Indiana University Press.

Kelman, H. C. (1973). Violence without moral restraint: Reflections on the dehumanization of victims and victimizers. *Journal of Social Issues, 29*(4), 25–61.

Leach, M. (1990). How to make use of technology. *Nursing, 44*(10), 7–12.

Levy, J. S., & Wachtel, P. L. (1979). Depersonalization: An effort at clarification. *The American Journal of Psychoanalysis, 38,* 291–300.

Mann, R. E. (1992). Preserving humanity in an age of technology. *Intensive and Critical Care Nursing, 8,* 54–59.

Merideth, C., & Edworthy, J. (1995). Are there too many alarms in the intensive care unit? An overview of the problems. *Journal of Advanced Nursing, 21,* 15–20.

Mitcham, C. (1994). *Thinking through technology: The path between engineering and philosophy.* Chicago: University of Chicago Press.

Purcell, C. (1994). *White heat: People and technology.* London: BBC Publications.

Raatikainen, R. (1989). Values and ethical principles in nursing. *Journal of Advanced Nursing, 14,* 92–96.

Reiser, S. J. (1978). *Medicine and the reign of technology.* Cambridge: Cambridge University Press.

Rudge, T. (1999). Situating wound management: Technoscience, dressings and "other" skins. *Nursing Inquiry, 6,* 167–177.

Sandelowski, M. (1988). A case of conflicting paradigms: Nursing and reproductive technology. *Advances in Nursing Science, 10*(3), 35–45.

Sandelowski, M. (1997). (Ir)Reconcilable differences? The debate concerning nursing and technology. *Image: Journal of Nursing Scholarship, 29*(2), 169–174.

Sandelowski, M. (1999). Troubling distinctions: A semiotics of the nursing/technology relationship. *Nursing Inquiry, 6,* 198–207.

Simpson, R. L., & Brown, L. N. (1985). High-touch/high-technology computer applications in nursing. *Nursing Administration Quarterly, 9*(4), 62–68.

Winner, L. (1977). *Autonomous technology.* Cambridge, MA: MIT Press.

Chapter 10

Suffering and Growth in the Shadow of Machines: Nursing and the Iron Lung, 1928–1955

Lynne H. Dunphy

The Man in the Iron Lung

I scream
The body electric
this yellow, metal, pulsating cylinder
Whooshing all day, all night
In its repetitious, dull mechanical rhythm.
Rudely it inserts itself in the map of my body,
which my midnight mind,
Dream drenched cartographer of terra incognita,
Draws upon the dark parchment of sleep.
I scream
In my body electric

Mark O'Brien

INTRODUCTION

In the first part of the twentieth century in America, the polio virus "leapfrogged" across the country, stopping who knew when or where, randomly, with no discernible pattern, wreaking havoc in its path (Black, 1996). Other diseases killed more than polio, but none was more feared. The crippling effects of the disease were apparent in the survivors; polio struck mainly the innocent—babies and children. The 1930s had a national incidence of 7,500 nationwide (a peak of 16,000 cases in 1931, and a dip in cases to 2,000 in 1938—confirming the sporadic and random nature of the epidemics); by the mid-1940s there were more than 40,000 cases on average per year, with an increasing number of cases affecting adults (Gould, 1995; Paul, 1971). With the advent of the Salk polio vaccine and mass immunization campaigns, the epidemics ceased, rather suddenly, by the mid-1950s (Cohn, 1955). Since that time, certainly in the nursing literature, there has been very little examination of nursing's role during the polio epidemics and the changes that emerged as a result. It is as though the memories of that time and those events have been closed up in big, black boxes, and put "under the bed," "up in the attic," anywhere where the devastatingly painful memories would be out of sight and mind. It is only recently, in a spurt of spring housecleaning, that we in nursing have discovered that black box, and having collectively blocked out what it contained, opened the cover (Dunphy, 2000).

This chapter argues that out of the terrible crisis of the polio epidemics, specifically as an outgrowth of "constant and relentless" care needed by patients in the iron lung, arose identifications of patients' need for caring. Additionally, I argue that the dynamics of the nurse–patient relationship arising in the context of the "machine" created a new and unique nexus for caring that has implications for the care of patients today.

"THE YELLOW CASKETS"

One of the fascinating things to emerge from the polio epidemics was the development of the iron lung. The idea of artificial ventilation had come about as early as the first part of the nineteenth century. A variety of devices and techniques were designed, most without success. Manual methods of artificial ventilation emerged, but there was no consistent, effective means of mechanical ventilation until 1928 (Magner, 1992; Porter, 1997). It was Dr. Phillip Drinker, an engineer at the Department of Ventilation and Illumination at the School of Public Health, Harvard University, who developed the first iron lung (Drinker & McKhann, 1986; Gould, 1995; Paul, 1971; Virtual Museum of the Iron Lung).

While observing his colleague Dr. Louis Shaw, a physiologist, measure the breathing of an anesthetized cat lying in a metal box with a rubber collar around its neck and its head exposed, Drinker had an idea. He curarized the breathing muscles of a cat, and placed its body, up to its neck, in a closed box, connected to a motor that pumped air into the box with a crude set of bellows. He was able to keep the cat alive for hours! Drinker and Shaw then constructed a human-sized respirator, utilizing the same principles as the "cat box." It consisted of a large, metal box, which opened and shut like a drawer, and had a rubber collar to fit around the neck of the patient to prevent any escape of air from the box (Drinker & McKhann, 1986; Gould, 1995; Paul, 1971).

Drinker's device was controversial. His brother Cecil, a Harvard professor of physiology, remained skeptical that the device could work. He thought that any collar tight enough to prevent the outflow of air would impede cerebral circulation. Drinker placed himself in the apparatus, proving its safety. Although not originally designed for any specific group of patients, those with polio seemed an ideal population upon which to demonstrate and test his machine (Bowen, 1970; Drinker & McKhann,1986; Paul, 1971; Wilson, 1944).

"A SUMMER PLAGUE"

"Fear hung like heat in the summer air," according to one source, referring to how the epidemic struck in late summer and early fall (Black, 1996, p. 30). The polio virus invaded the motor cells of the spinal cord and brain stem, preferring specifically the anterior horn cells, which send messages of movement to the skeletal muscles of the body—arms, legs, abdomen, chest, and neck. Ironically, and tragically, it left unaffected the dorsal sensory cells which receive incoming messages such as pain, temperature, balance, and vibration (Greteman, 1944; Kidd, 1943; Kottke & Kubicek, 1949). Thus, "if a hand . . . paralyzed by polio were placed on a hot stove burner, it would feel the heat through the healthy dorsal cells. But no matter how urgent the messages the brain sent to remove that hand, it would stay, flesh burning, the destroyed anterior cells unable to do their job of relaying the signals to the hand" (Black, 1996, p. 16).

Any combination of anterior horn cells could be affected, but legs were more often affected than arms, and the large muscles of the hands were more affected than the small ones. The disease usually began with a headache and flu-like symptoms, including a fever. Often, the disease was self-limiting, the sufferer not even aware that he or she had successfully battled the virus. But in other cases, paralysis occurred, sometimes within a few hours but more often over the course of two to three days, ending with the breaking of the fever. Any combination of muscles might be affected, including the intercostals and diaphragm, leading to extreme difficulty in breathing (Dowling, 1977; Kidd, 1943; Kottke & Kubicek, 1949; Muldar, 1998; Thompson, 1938).

Additionally, the virus could also affect the bulbar cells of the central nervous system, causing severe respiratory difficulties by another route. It could affect the cranial nerves that controlled eye and facial muscles, and interfered with chewing; more ominously, it could attack the cranial nerves that operate the pharynx, the soft palate, and larynx, making swallowing, breathing, and speaking difficult or impossible, endangering the lives of victims in yet another manner. In some cases, the virus ravaged the body of its victim with both spinal and bulbar paralysis. Treatment of the two types of paralysis often conflicted. The iron lung was most effective for persons with spinal paralysis, those cases where the patient's respiratory muscles were affected. The iron lung, ironically, posed great risks for patients with pharyngeal paralysis, and its usage was controversial. This group of patients could die flat on their backs, gurgling and aspirating on their own secretions. If the rhythm was not synchronized with their unaffected respiratory muscles, some patients fought the machine. And yet some were misdiagnosed and had been placed within the terrifying machine (Mendelson, Solomon, & Lindemann, 1958).

By the 1940s, bulbar polio, which resulted in pharyngeal paralysis, was treated with tracheotomies, although this too was to remain a controversial issue. With active nursing care, "constant and relentless"; by working with the patient to clear secretions through suctioning and postural drainage techniques; by quelling the patient's anxiety and avoiding panic; the patient might be eased through the pharyngeal paralysis, which might only last for a few days anyway. This would avoid the infection, bleeding, mucous plugs, and terror that could accompany the tracheotomy (Dowling, 1977; Greteman, 1944; Helling, 1941; Kidd, 1943; Kottke & Kubicek, 1949).

Kathryn Black describes her mother, Virginia, a polio victim in the early 1950s: A respirator's rhythmic *ka-thum-pa* sounds and the cacophony of mechanized, wheezing breath led them to Mother. The iron lung encased Virginia in a vacuum. Pumps worked at regular intervals applied first positive, then negative pressure, pushing on her lungs to expel air, then pulling on them to draw more in—an awkwardly consistent cadence. In this acute, dangerous stage of the disease, Mother likely lay semiconscious, unable to speak. One tube entered her nose, and another penetrated her neck. (Black, 1996, p. 14)

"SUCH COMFORT!"

For many patients, the lung provided blissful relief. Regina Woods wrote,

before I realized what was happening I was in a huge cylinder with only my head sticking out. A few adjustments were quickly made and it was closed. To my amazement, the cylinder had rolled open and it had not been necessary to stuff me through the small opening at the end. Such comfort! I was no longer struggling to breathe and the whole thing seemed simply wonderful. (1994, p. 14)

Not all accounts were so benign, however:

From what I could see, their faces above their masks were taut and strained, full of ugly determination. They lay me down between the jaws of a yawning box which had appeared from nowhere . . . yet a part of me remained detached, watching myself shout and struggle, shocked at my lack of my control . . . now my head was sinking backward to the floor; the whole box was being tilted.

Suddenly it came to me . . . this was a coffin and they were burying me alive. (Gould, 1995, p. 310)

HOSPITALS AND NURSING, 1928–1955

Although they were originally charity-based facilities for long-term care of the chronically ill, by the 1920s hospitals were firmly established as scientific facilities for acute medical interventions (Lynaugh, 1989). The size and number of hospitals increased dramatically, and their philanthropic ethos had already been modified to include a business sensibility (Rosenberg, 1987; Rosner, 1989). They began attracting middle-class, paying patients. Medical technology had come to play an important, even central role. X-rays and EKGs allowed doctors to literally "see" inside the human body. Anesthesiology and improved asepsis encouraged surgical intervention. Diagnostic laboratories allowed doctors to identify microbes, and by the 1940s they had added powerful antibiotics to their pharmacologic armeterium (Howell, 1989). Medicine continued to increase in stature, prestige, and power (Starr, 1982). The introduction of iron lung technology was yet another example of this trend.

The rise of the third-party payer system in the1930s provided support for increased hospital utilization. Graduate nurses, rather than student nurses, began to be used to provide care to increasingly sick hospital patients (Kalisch & Kalisch, 1995; Melosh, 1982; Reverby, 1985, 1987; Starr, 1982). This development was reinforced by the economic conditions of the Great Depression in the 1930s, (Kalisch & Kalisch, 1995; Reverby, 1987). Patients flocked to hospitals in the 1930s, perceiving them as charitable institutions; patients and families who had previously used private duty nurses employed in their homes were no longer able to afford them (Reverby, 1985). Out-of-work nurses were begging for employment and willing to accept the smallest wage offered by the hospitals along with room and board.

Studies over a number of years had supported the trend to a graduate nursing work force. It was beginning to be acknowledged that depending on a nursing student work force was not consistent with sound educational practices. The nurse leadership of the time, many of whom were both nursing educators and hospital administrators, supported this move (Melosh, 1982). Many nurse leaders saw the alignment of nursing with "science," represented in the "new" hospital centers with a graduate RN work force, as a strategy toward professionalization (Reverby, 1987).

POLIO NURSES: FOLLOWING THE EPIDEMICS

Nurses were integral to the care of patients with polio from the very beginning of the epidemics in the early part of the century, and the work was always dangerous. No one really understood how polio was transmitted from one person to another, so fear of contagion was present in the care of these patients from the very beginning. In the epidemic in New York City in 1916, one of the first major outbreaks in this country, over 72,000 cats were slaughtered in an attempt to cut down on the spread of the disease (Gould, 1995; Rogers, 1992). Panic, hysteria, confusion, and chaos characterized this time period, with quarantine as the predominant response; dying children were refused care. No one had any idea, however, how long the disease was contagious (Seavey, Smith, & Wagner, 1998). In subsequent outbreaks, it was not unheard of for student nurses to become ill; some died (anecdotal information, American Association for the History of Nursing [AAHN] conference, 1999). Nurses who had cared for polio patients during the time period under investigation were interviewed and asked about their fear. They reported the following:

Researcher: You mentioned that you had some fear of contracting polio?

Nurse Informant: Yeah, I think everybody did in those days, that was assigned to it . . . I mean, you had to gown up, you wore a mask, you did all that . . . I think there was greater fear of contracting polio than AIDs today . . . because you knew if you got it you could be crippled for life . . . during the infectious stage, nurses were afraid.

Juanita Howell, RN, talked about her work as a "polio" nurse. She recalls thinking, "Why don't I try the polio clinic? . . . They needed help, the patients were coming in from all around the state, nurses were coming from all over the country, it was just a very desperate time. . . . We had a number of nurses who came back from the war in 1945 and followed the epidemics" (Howell, 1998, p. 149). She remembers that the polio nurses wore street clothes to work because they were afraid of the reaction of average citizens who observed them in uniform getting off the bus and going into the polio clinic.

By the 1940s, along with the Red Cross, the National Foundation for Infantile Paralysis (NFIP) held regular training sessions for nurses in the care of polio patients, especially those in iron lungs. Large numbers of nurses attended regional workshops that brought the most up-to-date information to all nurses interested in learning the techniques of polio nursing. These nurses, often educators and supervisors, would return to their communities and provide training for local nurses. Additionally, since it was impossible to predict where the next outbreak would occur, or its severity, any community in need would be supplied with intensive, emergency training courses by representatives from the Red Cross and NFIP (Cohn, 1955; Seavey, Smith, & Wagner, 1998). Additionally, the Red Cross and the NFIP also maintained an active registry of "polio nurses" and provided support, including housing for those nurses, when epidemics struck. In some locales, the nurses lived in private homes secured by the Red Cross (Whitman, 1948). They were welcomed by the communities that they came to serve. As the number of patients who survived in iron lungs grew, respiratory centers that were dedicated to the care and rehabilitation of chronic patients popped up (Black, 1996; Cohn, 1955; Hamil, 1957; Weligoschek, 1950; Whitman, 1948).

In a 1938 article, Dr. T. Campbell Thompson noted, "In no disease, except perhaps pneumonia, is expert nursing care so essential. Rest, complete and prolonged, mental and physical, is by far the single most important factor in aiding the poisoned motor cells of the spinal cord to recover" (Thompson, 1938, p. 145). Prevention of pneumonia, breakdown of skin areas, and physiologic changes resulting from the patient's severe restriction of movement were all designated as important nursing responsibilities associated with respirator care (Dunphy, 2000).

NURSING AND THE IRON LUNG

The iron lung was the first machine that was able to keep a human being alive; and who was it who cared for the patient in the machine? Why, it was the nurses, of course! One article of the time makes the following point: "Professor Drinker has stressed more than once the fact that, even if a respirator works perfectly, it will not take the place of nursing care" (Norcross, 1939, p. 1067).

The physical management of the patient in the iron lung was a challenge. This was identified early in its development. J. L. Wilson, M.D., helped Drinker refine his early respirator. He describes the care of the second patient to be put into the lung, a strapping young man:

He seemed almost totally paralyzed and the use of the respirator demonstrated several things. One, the great difficulty of caring for a big man. The thing was closed with multiple clamps on a hard rubber gasket so there was no access to the man's body to clean him or do anything to him. (Wilson, 1971)

Wilson noted that it took a heroic effort, with six men and nurses in an organized team, to bathe him. This led Wilson, on the advice of Philip Drinker, to buy some portholes made for boats and have them welded onto the machine so that they could be opened. They then fitted the portholes with rubber collars through which hands could be inserted to "manipulate" the patient without taking him out of the tank and disturbing his respirations. The work of prioritizing nursing care was clearly laid out (Dunphy, 2000; Paul, 1971).

NURSING CARE: THE MASTER OF THE MACHINE

Just as does the critical care nurse of today, the nurse caring for a patient in an iron lung had to learn every aspect of handling the machine (and hence, the patient *in* the machine). One article reviewed provides the heading, "The patient is a person—the respirator is a machine, the nurse must understand both to give effective care to the respirator patient" (Parisi, 1951, p. 360). The negative pressure of the machine was usually set somewhere between 14 and 18 respirations per minute, which was accomplished by turning a wheel near the motor. Additionally, the pressure within the lung had to be set, controlling the important depth of respirations, estimated between 10 and 20 cm of water pressure, indicated by a pressure gauge. It was the physician who was responsible for determining the depth and rate of respiration, usually based on the size and condition of the patient, type of lung used, and the like. However, sources note that it fell to the nurse to monitor the breathing of the patient and make whatever adjustments were necessary (nurse informants; Harmer & Henderson, 1939, 1955; NFIP procedure guides, 1949; Price, 1954; Tracy, 1949).

The nurse, as master of the machine, had the important responsibility of adapting it to the individual patient. The nurse had to be attuned to the patient's every breath, to any small sign of distress, or change in color. The nurse had to be prepared to suction, apply oxygen, adjust the tilt of the machine to facilitate drainage (this could be done), or call the physician when a tracheotomy needed to be performed:

The care of the polio respirator patient is tremendous responsibility. It is physically exhausting in actual physical energy expended to care for the patient, and it is a mental strain trying to imbue him with confidence and a hopeful outlook. It is a great strain also watching for signs indicating a change (adverse) in the patient's condition. (Manfreda, 1991, p. 7)

The nurse provided the important human link between patient and machine, and thus, between life and death. The life of the patient in the iron lung was always in the nurse's hands.

One of the biggest mental responsibilities is remembering to check on the respirator pressure. Pressure may be lost from the smallest leak occurring around the head opening, a porthole door being left open, incomplete closure of the head and body parts of the respirator, or an unplugged opening, such as the opening designed to admit intravenous tubing. A patient's life could be lost from pressure failure. (Manfreda, 1991, p. 7)

Every nurse spoke of the mental stress of having to be prepared for power failures. "Once the current on three of the respirators failed. Until maintenance could restore it, we had to man the respirator bellow by hand. This is extremely hard to do, the person pumping tiring within a minute or two" (Manfreda, 1991, p. 7). Teamwork in this situation was also essential for the patient's survival. One nurse informant shared the following: "The staff on duty (doctors, nurses, orderlies), in short, everybody available and able, lined up and in relays we kept the respirator going." Another nurse informant stated that her greatest fear was: "Power failures. And there was never enough help. Those were the days that I recall working twelve plus hours per day. Without a day off for weeks on end." A similar comment was given by another "polio" nurse: "someone had to provide the manual power. The machines could be switched into manual and operated by hand. There was a crank on the back of it, and maintenance people, gardeners, sweepers—anyone who was available came to help" (Howell, 1989, p. 151).

There was a flip side to "mastery of the machine." The machine gave nurses tremendous control over their patients. The following quote is from Regina Woods, just one of many examples in the patient literature on being in an iron lung that records episodes of cruelty on the part of caregivers:

Various ways were tried to get those and those like me out of the lungs that lined the halls like so many yellow caskets, their motionless inhabitants filled with fear and rage. Fear they would not survive the next attempt to help them and rage that they could do nothing to strike back when the keepers went beyond the bounds of human decency. (Woods, 1994, p. 18)

The following incident was recollected by Marilyn Rogers, nine years old in 1949 and in an iron lung when this occurred:

I had a cloth around my neck, to keep my neck from getting rubbed away by the collar . . . one day it slid . . . I couldn't breathe. I was crying and calling the nurse. You had to learn to really melt to get her attention. She came in and seemed really frustrated, overworked, and just too busy. So I told her what was wrong and she told me to stop crying. She said she would turn my respirator off if I didn't stop crying. When she did, I passed out immediately. (Rogers, 1998, p. 27)

A patient informant recalled:

I really have no complaints except there was one nurse at night when the collar, the pad around my neck . . . would slip and I'd have to call her and she knew I could not breathe and she would open the respirator and take the collar off and then go down the hall and get the diaper and then go into the hole and get a pad and all the while I am not breathing. So she'd come back and she'd slowly fold it and finally get it and powder it and finally get it around my neck and then put me back in. God I used to hate that lady because she kept me out there for so long.

It is only fair to recall that numerous stories of wonderful experiences with nurses abound—warm, funny, brave nurses persevering bravely in the face of great difficulties.

SHARED POWERLESSNESS

Interviews with nurses were revealing (Dunphy, 2000). One recalled a young woman she had cared for—a "chronic," that is, beyond the acute stages of her illness, but still iron lung dependent. Our informant was a student nurse at the time, and on her pediatric rotation. "And being at that hospital, supposedly learning my pediatric experience, this being an adult, it was like this isn't fair! I'm being used! . . . and we really felt we were being dumped on! But immaturity was part of our problem too." Another nurse informant continued to reflect on this patient. She recalled, "she wanted to be waited on constantly. And then I had the frustration of not being able to care for my other patients. And being a young nurse, I couldn't comprehend why she was being so demanding." Reflecting on this situation today, she explained that at the time she didn't interpret the behavior as the anxiety she could now see clearly that it was but rather that she was a "selfish" individual. "I wasn't mature enough to understand what she was going through."

Another nurse informant told us, "The psychological needs were so vital and yet we didn't attach as much importance to those things in those years as we do today. . . . We weren't as empathic. We weren't as understanding." She spoke of the need "for better understanding" and concluded with the statement, "We were so harassed with keeping our patients alive and working the hours that we did, and having our own frustrations that we couldn't do more than we were doing, and seeing this never ending admission of patients."

PSYCHOLOGICAL MILIEU

The emotional needs of patients with polio frequently went unacknowledged by all the professionals involved, certainly not just by nurses (Davis, 1963; Gould, 1995). Doctors seldom touched patients, and when they did it was with gloved hands. Some doctors did not even enter the rooms of children with polio, but stood in the doorway or waved through a glass partition. One doctor recalled, "You wanted to pick them up and hold them [the children], but you just didn't do that" (Whitfield, 1994, p. 18). When staff did enter the rooms, they came covered in gowns and masks, which they shed when they left (usually as soon as possible).

Doris Seligman, a teenager in 1949 when she was stricken with polio, recalls that she lay "encased in an iron lung and isolated except for some rare contact with nurses . . . soaked in urine most of the time" (Black, 1996, p. 67). It was not until a night when the hospital lost electrical power and someone rushed to hand pump her iron lung that she realized she was not forgotten.

During the 1930s, very little attention was paid to the psychosocial side of patient care (Barbour, 1932; Prugh & Tagiuri, 1954). Children were separated from parents and those who became excessively anxious were viewed as overattached to their mothers, consistent with the psychoanalytic views of the day. Parents who were perceived as excessively anxious were labeled "psychologically immature." During the acute phase of the illness, families were only allowed to visit once a week in most settings, and for a very brief period. It was theorized that children would make a "better adjustment" to their illness this way. They were being prepared for the long road ahead to recovery (Fairchild, 1952; Seavey, Smith, & Wagner, 1998). Nurses were cautioned to not be too sympathetic to the children, that an "objective" [read: professional] attitude was to be maintained at all times.

A 1935 *New England Journal of Medicine* article stated that for a child who had completely recovered, "the disease seems to have no darker memory than an attack of measles" (Barbour, 1935, p. 565). Another source boldly asserted, "No crippled individual should be left to indulge in his own thoughts" (Kidd, 1943). One source from 1937 argued that the hospitalized child should be surrounded by an atmosphere of "neutrality"; it was thought better to have no visitors than to have anxious families and friends hovering nearby (Harmison, 1935).

A survey of nursing school curricula and nursing textbooks shows little attention to the nurse–patient relationship prior to the 1950s. Journal articles do acknowledge the need to "remember the patient" in the lung and to individualize care. Actual methods of facilitating communications and in-depth discussion of the psychological needs of the patients were not found in the nursing journals and texts surveyed (Dunphy, 2000). Statements such as the following set the tone: "Nursing care must, of course, be adapted to the particular needs of the patient. The initial fear of the machine, the restriction of motion, and later, anxiety over the removal from the respirator all present psychological problems"(Harmer & Henderson, 1955, p. 795). The text then goes on in greater detail to discuss the physical care of the patient.

A CALL FOR CARING

A 1947 article by Morton Seidenfeld, Ph.D., Director of Psychological Services, National Foundation for Infantile Paralysis, New York City, began to sound a different voice in the nursing literature. In the article, entitled "Psychological Considerations in Poliomyelitis Care," Seidenfeld (1947) clearly identifies listening to the patient, and learning about the patient as an individual as priorities of nursing care: "Give him a chance to 'get it off his chest,' " he counsels. "Sure, it will take time. Sure, you are busy with a dozen other youngsters on the ward. But don't forget that this *is* nursing care and to Johnny [the metaphorical patient] it may be more calming in its effects than phenobarbital and more lasting in its values" (p. 369). Seidenfeld (1948, 1955) says the whole process of listening is part of a preventive mental hygiene plan that may avert more severe tensions.

The care and concern that the nurses felt for their patients comes through as clearly in accounts as reports of cruelty and indifference. One nurse discussed some of what they did with the children while they were in the hospital:

We read to them. And we would push their beds all together for entertainment. . . . In the winter when it snowed we'd pull all the beds to the window. In fact, we'd go out on the big porches and make snowballs and bring it in so the children could hold the snowballs. . . . And if anyone had a birthday, why, there was a big party. We'd have a cake and candles. (Tafil, 1998, pp. 35–36)

She talked about how every ward had a big room that they could pull the beds to, like a living room. One patient was asked what was going through her head, at age nine, "being on the machine." The following is her response:

Staying alive. The staff was very, very nice to us. Some of the nurses that they called "plague nurses" at the National Foundation, they were the best. One of them brought peas in with straws so that we could see if we could hit the ceiling to increase our vital capacity. I usually give nicknames to everybody. She wore purple fingernail polish. So I called her "Purple." (Rogers, 1998, p. 26)

CONCLUSIONS

Clearly, it was nurses who were most instrumental in the implementation of this radical new technology, the iron lung. The brave and resourceful nurses who cared for the patients in iron lungs became technologically proficient "masters of the machine," while attempting to integrate traditional nursing values of caring and individualizing care. However, often the goals of keeping their patients alive and attending to multiple physiological needs, compounded by large numbers of very ill patients during the epidemics, appropriately, took precedence. The prevailing psychological mores of the day, especially in the early days of the epidemics, did not support sensitivity to the emotional needs of patients and families. Although psychological approaches were to become more enlightened during the late 1940s and 1950s, these ideas were yet to be mainstreamed into nursing curricula. Young nurses, and student nurses in particular, were not always prepared to meet the overwhelming emotional needs of patients in iron lungs. Students continued to be "used" for service needs, with not enough time and support to provide the high level of care that these patients needed.

The constant and relentless care rendered by nurses caring for patients in iron lungs in the first half of the twentieth century demonstrated technological mastery predicated on intimate sensitivity to their patients' physiological needs and changes. It was up to them to make the decision regarding adjusting the pressures, suctioning, calling the doctor to perform a tracheotomy, or soothing the anxiety of the patient with pharyngeal paralysis. Aspects of this care also cast light on less savory aspects of nursing practice, in the form of episodes of insensitivity, even cruelty. Historian Thomas Olson argues that "handling, controlling, and managing" abilities of nursing students were what were valued between the years 1915 and 1937, that the "language of caring" was absent (Olson, 1987, p. 117; Rinker, 2000, pp. 133–134). This inquiry unfolded tales of knowledgeable, committed, brave, and creative nurses confronted with overwhelmingly ill patients, many of them infants and children, frightening and new technology, low pay and work in hospital structures where they were largely powerless (Grando, 2000). Margaret Sandelowski (1999) notes, "Specialty nursing practices built around technologies remaining in medical jurisdiction serve primarily the interests of organized medicine and hospitals" (p. 61). In essence, the physicians "controlled" the lungs, in that they ordered the lung, set the pressures; and the nurses were often students, young and educated to prioritize physiological needs over psychological ones, often contrary to their own caring instincts. An interview with a physician who had cared for polio patients during the epidemics revealed the following memories:

The acute polio wards, when new cases came in, were in an old building. There were big, open wards, maybe only one or two private rooms for some of the worst infectious diseases. And of course there was always the sound of the respirators: whoosh . . . whoosh . . . whoosh . . . whoosh. The sound of the machines for suctioning. Those that had tracheotomies would develop phlegm in their mouths—more like a gurgling sound. And I remember the sight of the physical therapists and the nurses coming around trying to position arms and legs. (Affeldt, 1998, p. 137)

The care of patients with polio, especially those in iron lungs, was overwhelming and traumatic for caretakers as well as patients. The care was "constant and relentless." Often the patient's very life hung in the balance. There was shared suffering by patients and caretakers. But out of suffering comes growth. Patients lived who might have died. Technological proficiencies developed out of necessity and invention; and there was also an identification of the importance of caring in the relationship between patient and nurse, an ethos that was to become more fully developed in the latter part of the twentieth century.

REFERENCES

Affeldt, J. (1998). Interview. In G. Seaveyina, J. S. Smith, & P. Wagner (Eds.), *A paralyzing fear* (pp. 135–146). New York: TV Books.

Barbour, E. H. (1932). Social aspects of poliomyelitis. *New England Journal of Medicine, 207,* 1195–1196.

Barbour, E. H. (1935). Adjustment during the four years of patients handicapped by poliomyelitis. *New England Journal of Medicine, 213,* 563–565.

Black, K. (1996). *In the shadow of polio.* Reading, MA: Addison-Wesley.

Bowen, C. D. (1970). *Family portraits.* New York: Scribner's.

Cohn, V. (1955). *Four billion dimes.* Minneapolis, MN: Minneapolis Star and Tribune.

Davis, F. (1963). *Passage through crisis.* Indianapolis, IN: Bobbs-Merrill.

Dowling, H. (1977). *Fighting infection: Conquests of the twentieth century.* Cambridge, MA: Harvard University Press.

Drinker, P., & McKhann, C. (1986). The iron lung: First practical means of respiratory support. *Journal of the American Medical Association, 255,* 1476–1481.

Dunphy, L. M. (2000). The steel cocoon: Tales of the nurses and patients of the iron lung. *Nursing History Review, 9* (in press).

Fairchild, L. M. (1952). Some psychological factors observed in poliomyelitis patients. *American Journal of Physical Medicine, 31,* 275–281.

Gould, T. (1995). *A summer plague: Polio and its survivors.* New Haven, CT: Yale University Press.

Grando, V. (2000). A hard day's work: Institutional nursing in the post–WWII era. *Nursing History Review 8,* 169–184.

Greteman, T. J. (1944). Nursing care of acute poliomyelitis. *American Journal of Nursing, 44*(10), 929–933.

Harmer, B. (1936). *Textbook of the principles and practices of nursing* (3rd ed.). New York: Macmillan.

Harmer, B., & Henderson, V. (1939). *Textbook of the principles and practices of nursing* (4th ed.). New York: Macmillan.

Harmer, B., & Henderson, V. (1955). *Textbook of the principles and practices of nursing* (5th ed.). New York: Macmillan.

Harmison, B. (1935). Nursing care of a child in the respirator. *American Journal of Nursing, 35*(5), 479–481.

Helling, H. (1941). The patient in the respirator. *American Journal of Nursing, 41*(11), 1322–1324.

Howell, J. (1989). Machines and medicine: Technology transforms the American hospital. In D. Long & J. Golden (Eds.), *The American general hospital*. Ithaca, NY: Cornell University Press.

Howell, J. (1998). Interview. In N. G. Seavey, J. S. Smith, & P. Wagner (Eds.), *A paralyzing fear* (pp. 147–152). New York: TV Books.

Kalisch, P., & Kalisch, B. (1995). *The history of American nursing*. Philadelphia: Lippincott.

Kidd, D. B. (1943). *The physical treatment of anterior poliomyelitis*. London: Faber & Faber.

Kottke, F. J., & Kubicek, W. G. (1949). The care of the patient with bulbar-respiratory poliomyelitis. *American Journal of Nursing, 49*(6), 374–378.

Lynaugh, J. (1989). From respectable domesticity to medical efficiency: The changing Kansas City Hospital, 1875–1920. In D. E. Long & J. Golden (Eds.), *The American general hospital* (pp. 21–39). Ithaca, NY: Cornell University Press.

Magner, L. (1992). *A history of medicine*. New York: Marcel Dekker.

Manfreda, E. (1991). Polio nursing: An abbreviated report to the Wallingford Chapter of the American Red Cross on my experience as a polio nurse in Akron, Ohio, August–October, 1952. *American Association for the History of Nursing Bulletin, 30*, 6–8.

Melosh, B. (1982). *The physician's hand: Work culture and conflict in American nursing*. Philadelphia: Temple University Press.

Mendelson, I., Solomon, P., & Lindemann, E. (1958). Hallucinations of poliomyelitis patients during treatment in a respirator. *Journal of Nervous and Mental Diseases, 126*, 421–428.

Muldar, D. (1998). Clinical observations on acute poliomyelitis. *Annals of the New York Academy of Sciences*, 1–10.

National Foundation for Infantile Paralysis (NFIP). (1949). *Negative pressure procedure book*. New York: NFIP & NLNE.

Norcross, M. F. (1939). The Drinker respirator. *American Journal of Nursing, 39*(10), 1063–1068.

O'Connor, B. (1948). Leading the fight on poliomyelitis. *Public Health Nursing, 34*(1), 12–16.

Olson, T. (1987). Caring or uncaring? *Nursing Outlook, 76*, 55–87.

Parisi, C. (1951). The patient in the respirator. *American Journal of Nursing, 51*(6), 360–363.

Paul, J. R. (1971). *A history of poliomyelitis*. New Haven, CT: Yale University Press.

Porter, R. (1997). *The greatest benefit to mankind*. New York: HarperCollins.

Price, A. L. (1954). *The art and science and spirit of nursing*. Philadelphia: W. B Saunders.

Prugh, D., & Tagiuri, C. K. (1954). Emotional aspects of the respirator care of patients with poliomyelitis. *Psychosomatic Medicine, 16*, 104–128.

Reverby, S. (1985). The search for the hospital yardstick: Nursing & the rationalization of hospital work. In J. W. Leavitt & R. Numbers (Eds.), *Sickness and health in America* (pp. 206–218). Madison: University of Wisconsin Press.

Reverby, S. (1987). *Ordered to care: The dilemma of American nursing, 1873–1945*. Cambridge, MA: Harvard University Press.

Rinker, S. (2000). To cultivate a feeling of confidence: The nursing of obstetric patients, 1890–1940. *Nursing History Review, 8*, 117–142.

Robinson, H. A., Finesinger, J. E., & Bierman, J. S. (1956). Psychiatric considerations in the adjustment of patients with poliomyelitis. *New England Journal of Medicine, 254*(21), 975–980.

Rogers, M. (1998). Interview. In N. G. Seavey, J. S. Smith, & P. Wagner (Eds.), *A paralyzing fear* (pp. 25–34). New York: TV Books.

Rogers, N. (1992). *Dirt and disease: Polio before FDR*. New Brunswick, NJ: Rutgers University Press.

Rosenberg, C. (1987). *The care of strangers*. New York: Basic Books.

Rosner, D. (1989). Doing well or doing good: The ambivalent focus of hospital administration. In D. E. Long & J. Golden (Eds.), *The American general hospital* (pp. 157–169). Ithaca, NY: Cornell University Press.

Sandelowski, M. (1999). Venous envy: The post–WWII debate over IV nursing. *Advances in Nursing Science, 22*(1), 52–62.

Seavey, N. G., Smith, J. S., & Wagner, P. (Eds). (1998). *A paralyzing fear: The triumph over polio in America*. New York: TV Books.

Seidenfeld, M. A. (1947). The psychological considerations in poliomyelitis care. *American Journal of Nursing, 47*(6), 369–370.

Seidenfeld, M. A. (1948). The psychological sequelae of poliomyelitis in children. *Nervous Child, 1*, 14–28.

Seidenfeld, M. A. (1955). Psychological implications of breathing difficulties in poliomyelitis. *American Journal of Orthopsychiatry, 25*, 788–801.

Starr, P. (1982). *The transformation of American medicine*. New York: Basic Books.

Tafil, E. (1998). Interview. In N. G. Seavey, J. S. Smith, & P. Wagner (Eds.), *A paralyzing fear* (pp. 35–38). New York: TV Books.

Thompson, C. T. (1938). The essential features of poliomyelitis. *Public Health Nursing, 30*, 142–147.

Tracy, M. A. (1949). *Nursing: An art and a science*. St. Louis, MO: Mosby.

Virtual Museum of the Iron Lung. Http://members.xoom.com/XOOM/lung museum/welcome.htm.

Visotsky, H. M., Hamburg, D. A., Goss, M. E., & Lebovits, B. Z. (1961). Coping behavior under extreme stress: Observations of patients with severe poliomyelitis. *Archives of General Psychiatry, 5*, 27–33.

Whitfield, T. J. (1994). Interview with Kathryn Black, cited in Black, K. (1996). *In the shadow of polio*. Reading, MA: Addison Wesley.

Weligoschek, J. (1950, February). Personal experience with polio. *Trained Nurse*, 68–74.

Whitman, T. (1948, June). The polio nurse: A personal account. *Trained Nurse*, 51–52.

Wilson, J. L. (1944). The use of the respirator. *Journal of the American Medical Association, 117*(6), 278–279.

Wilson, J. L. (1971). Memoirs of the development of the respirator. Unpublished memoirs. In J. Paul, *A history of poliomyelitis* (pp. 324–334). New Haven, CT: Yale University Press.

Woods, R. (1994). *Tales from the iron lung and how I got out of it*. Philadelphia: University of Pennsylvania Press.

Chapter 11

The Symbiosis of Technology and Caring: Nursing of Older Adults

Rebecca A. Johnson

INTRODUCTION

"That as we enjoy great advantages from the inventions of others, we should be glad of an opportunity to serve others by any invention of ours; and this we should do freely and generously" (Franklin, 1966, p. 144). The words of one of America's premier inventors and wisdom purveyors, Benjamin Franklin, provide insight into the issue of how technology and caring may combine to benefit older adults.

Technological advances have made it possible for people to live longer and healthier lives with each succeeding generation. These advancements created numerous related ethical issues in nursing and health care. One such issue is whether or not it is appropriate to extend life beyond the ability of the patient to enjoy it. Another issue is to what extent technological advances may be "rationed" in the drive for economical, cost-efficient health care delivery. The ultimate question may well be, to what extent do technological advances actually improve quality of life for the patient? Among older adults, the fastest growing segment of society worldwide, these questions become increasingly salient as older persons gradually face declining functional ability leading to dependence and, ultimately, death.

As health care becomes increasingly driven by technology in diagnostic assessment, treatment, monitoring of patients' responses to treatment, and rehabilitation to former levels of functioning, it has become necessary to continually revisit these issues, which are relevant to technology and health care. Nurses are expressly situated as frontline caregivers to raise these issues. If technology is viewed as the "invention of others" that Franklin discussed, what is "the invention of ours" that nurses should "give freely and generously"?

It seems that caring is the invention of nursing. It is both the moral ideal as described by Watson (1985), and the act of connecting with and assisting patients in ways that recognize and protect their dignity and humanity. The ways in which nurses connect with and assist patients are myriad, reflecting technological advances, psychomotor skills, and interpersonal relations. Locsin (1995) posited that technologically competent nursing practice occurs when nurses use machine technology grounded in the perspective of "Nursing As Caring." Thus nursing has the potential, as Benjamin Franklin advised, to enjoy great advantage from the invention of others while still giving freely of our own invention.

Clearly, nursing would not have advanced to its present level of nursing knowledge and expertise without the benefit of technological discoveries and inventions. As recently as the 1930s, nurses were expected to remove plants from patients' hospital rooms at night because they were believed to consume oxygen needed for healing. Nurses, when given the raw materials of cotton wadding and gauze, were also commonly found making wound dressings. Advances in technology and nursing knowledge have enabled nurses to place greater emphases on assessing and caring for patients' needs with an impressively high degree of sophistication. However, the perspective of caring has remained integral to nursing patients effectively. As technological inventions have advanced, the perspective of caring has become even more important, as nurses help patients and their families on a daily basis to grapple with ethically challenging decisions involving technology.

OLDER ADULTS AS RECIPIENTS OF NURSING'S INVENTION

Older adults are well acquainted with the importance of the nurse–patient relationship as a facilitator of their health. Nurses constantly employ their advanced communication skills to routinely manage the complexities of older adults' physical, psychosocial, and spiritual needs. Caring is the foundation of these exchanges. Meeting the older adult patient's expectations of the nurse–patient relationship is not possible if the exchange is not grounded in a caring perspective. The skills that nurses employ in viewing older adults holistically and within their own particular contexts demand a high level of caring. Given the challenges of the current health care environment, nurse caring becomes all important if sensitive assessments are to be the basis for careful diagnosis, intervention, and coordination of the many services needed by older adults with varying degrees of disability. The work of nurse practitioners and other advanced practice nurses cannot be effective if not conducted from a caring perspective. This is nursing's invention.

Historically, older adults and their families have relied on nurses to learn what they needed to know in order to prevent illness, and to manage illness and recovery. This teaching and learning must have occurred within an atmosphere of caring. Nurses freely shared their invention each time they offered consolation, information, and advice to their older adult patients. Thus, older adults have traditionally benefited from nursing's invention and nurses have benefited in return by achieving the coveted status of trusted, preferred caregiver. This trust relationship implies that all dimensions of the nursing invention will be employed to maximize health and independence among older adult patients. The nursing invention of caring may involve the therapeutic use of self or the therapeutic use of agents and technology to achieve mutual goals. Older adults are thus receptive to, and benefit from, nursing's invention.

OLDER ADULTS: CONSUMERS AND BENEFICIARIES OF TECHNOLOGICAL INVENTIONS

Older adults entering the twenty-first century have witnessed an astounding and historically unprecedented array of technological advances. This has been compounded with each group of successively older adults. For example, hallmark inventions encountered by those young-old (65–75 years of age) include development of nuclear technology in the 1940s and use of its power in deployment of nuclear weapons, utilities, and medical diagnosis; introduction of the television, computers, and advanced telecommunication techniques. The middle-old (76–85 years of age) have not only witnessed these inventions, but also the widespread delivery of electricity and public transportation to rural areas, introduction of mass communication, and the ability to destroy bacteria with antibiotics. However, the oldest-old (86 years and older—the fastest growing group) have experienced the greatest number of inventions since the turn of the twentieth century, including the automobile, the telephone, and the airplane, as well as widespread acceptance of germ theory and the mechanization of commerce and industry. Thus, older adults have been adapting to technological inventions not only for a much longer period, but also have been integrating a greater and more complex array of technological inventions than have today's younger adults. The baby boomers may actually be "invention lightweights" when one considers the extent to which the inventions experienced by older adults altered day-to-day life and the growth of society.

Older adults have also witnessed and benefited from considerable advances in health care during their lifetimes. Some of the oldest older adults, as sick children, may have received prescribed feeding formulas from china invalid feeders (vessels shaped like small cream pitchers through which nurses poured feedings into the patients' mouths). This technology required that the patient be alert, be able to suck and to swallow. These same oldest-old may now witness their great-grandchildren born at less than 20 weeks of age and being tube fed breast milk in a neonatal intensive care unit, their vital functions monitored and supported via nursing and technological inventions.

Anecdotal evidence supports that older adults are both astounded by and grateful for the advances in health care made possible by technological inventions. They have benefited from technology more than their parents and grandparents by living longer, healthier lives, and by having a greater chance to survive the illnesses that befall them. Older adults' considerable experience with technological invention predisposes them to accept that technological advancement is unending, although sometimes incomprehensible in magnitude and speed of development.

Technology Receptivity and Use

The argument might be advanced that because older adults have witnessed and greatly benefited from the advancement of technology, they are largely receptive to technology in general and in their own lives. The alternative point of view is just as easily taken that older adults are unreceptive to and fearful of technology. However, neither point of view has been adequately studied. Generally speaking, research has not supported negative stereotypes of older adults as being too reticent or technologically incompetent to accept "modern" advances (Weill, Rosen, & Wugalter, 1990).

Several reasons for additional study exist. Older adults may be less likely to be receptive to computerized technology because of a perceived dehumanizing effect (Czaja & Sharit, 1998). In an example of commonplace technology applicable to daily life, older adults were found to be significantly less likely to use automated teller machines (ATMs) than younger adults. Those who did were more likely to use a wider variety of other technologies, have more experience and feel more comfortable with computers. Older adults who avoided ATMs reported that they did so because of their fear for safety, or their discomfort associated with having no human contact in effecting their banking transactions (Rogers et al., 1996).

Using this same technology, previous research shows that those older adults with higher mechanical reasoning skills were more likely to use ATMs. Those who did not use them expressed more negative attitudes toward ATMs. Conversely, among older adults who did not use ATMs, those who had tried an ATM expressed more positive attitudes than those who had not (Smither & Braun, 1994).

The findings regarding attitudes of older adults toward computers seem to suggest that, given adequate experience and training, older adults may be no less receptive nor less likely to use them than younger adults. However, the chronological context for older adults must be considered. Most had no opportunity to learn about computers while they were in school and computers were not commonly used in the workplace before they retired. Thus, fewer older adults were trained in use of computers associated with their work. This may contribute to the findings that older adults are less receptive to computers and less likely to use them. In a study by Marquie, Thon, and Baracat (1994), older office workers were found to have more fear, anxiety, and negative computer attitudes. They also had less computer training than younger counterparts. Other investigators found that older workers had less confidence in independently problem solving a computer-based error than younger workers (Birdi & Zapf, 1997). Older workers were more likely to use written documentation than to ask others for assistance. Evidence suggests that it may be the quick response of computers that produces anxiety for older adults (Laguna & Babcock, 1997). For example, older adults were found to have significantly higher computer anxiety than younger adults. However, their anxiety was not related to errors that they made while completing tasks using the computer but to their perceived lack of decision time in working and solving problems with the computer.

Although it is difficult to ascertain the sequencing of anxiety and lack of training, research has shown that older adults' attitudes toward computers improved with positive learning experiences (Baldi, 1997). Thus, it may be concluded that the type of training and experiences that older adults undergo with computers influences their receptivity. It may also be concluded that older adults may need more training sessions than younger adults.

Indeed, some research has shown that older adults' attitudes toward computers were modifiable with training and experience (Czaja & Sharit, 1998). Key factors influencing their attitudes included their comfort with computers, their perceived efficacy, dehumanization, and control over computers. The influence of gender was also revealed. For example, after a six-week training course on word processing, older women had less positive attitudes toward computers than did older men; more computer experience was associated with more positive attitudes and with learning more word processing knowledge. It was notable that after this six-week course, subjects tended to like computers less than before the course. In a related finding, Temple and Gavillet (1990) found that after a 12-hour computer course, there was no decrease in computer anxiety, although subjects' computer literacy was significantly improved.

Thus, it is apparent that type of exposure and learning may influence older adults' attitudes toward computers (Dyck & Smither, 1996). Others have reported that attitudes toward computers improved in older adults with brief training sessions (Kelley et al., 1999). Study of older adults' continued use of an electronic bulletin board showed that the most important predictor of computer anxiety was degree of success at initial training—education and income were not predictive, as was reported in other national samples (Kelley et al., 1999). It may be surmised that the combination of ample positive experience and short training courses may help to allay anxiety. Dyck and Smither (1994) previously found that older adults had less computer anxiety and had more positive attitudes toward computers than younger adults, despite the fact that they had less experience and less computer confidence overall. However, those older adults with higher experience levels had lower computer anxiety levels and more positive attitudes toward computers.

Several factors have stimulated computer software designers to devote considerable study to ways of making software more compatible with older adults' needs (Hutchison, Eastman, & Tirrito, 1997). These include awareness that older adults' competence and attitudes toward computers are amenable to change, the fact that they comprise the fastest growing demographic group, and anticipation of the baby boomers' aging (many of whom may be very experienced with computers and other forms of technocommunication). Aging and technological inventions are also a combination of interest to health care providers trying to meet the needs of this group. The challenge exists in the fact that older adults are a diverse group with varying levels of techno-receptivity. Use of technology in helping to maintain older adults' independence may gradually become commonplace.

Use of Helping Technologies

Helping technologies may have an especially important role to play because of the mobility of society and the geographic distances between many older adults and their families. The goal of helping technologies is to maximize independence and functioning among those with disabilities.

Restoring and maintaining functioning via the assistance of technology is the central focus of rehabilitation engineering. This profession has been in existence for many years and has resulted in considerable help for the elderly (Coombs, 1994). One example of helping technologies used in rehabilitation includes strength training and visual feedback to regain muscle mass. Postural stability is enhanced and falls are prevented. Another example is development and application of a wandering alert device, worn on the ankle or wrist of patients with dementia who are known to wander. The device sounds an alarm when the older adult passes a sensor, moving beyond designated locations in long-term care facilities. This type of technology increases the safety of older adults and enhances the vigilance of caregivers. Assurance of safety is an increasingly heavier burden with reduced staffing and increased nurse–patient ratios.

Dibner (1990) summarized findings on personal emergency response systems (PRS) and reported another helping technology for older adults. It is interesting to note that, even in 1990, sufficient research had been done to enable a substantive literature review. The findings showed that PRS greatly reduced anxiety of older adults living alone, and lessened the stress of their family members. This early literature review analyzed nine studies documenting the users of PRS (women in their late seventies and early eighties, living alone, with multiple disabilities). On the whole, users reported that their health had improved since they began using PRS, even though they became more frail over a year's usage period. They also reported less dizziness, fewer feelings of vulnerability, and generally felt better about themselves with an increased sense of security. Anecdotal reports of friends and neighbors of older adults who used PRS showed that they believed that PRS changed the users' lives by increasing their independence and helping to allay their anxiety about being alone. Studies are needed to ascertain the effect of PRS on health services' use and role in preventing and shortening hospital stays. However, PRS have been associated with use of fewer support services, such as physical therapy, homemaking services, and mobile meals (Ruchlin & Morris, 1981). Thus, PRS have had rapid acceptance among older adults and their families.

While PRS may facilitate independence and security by providing a "lifeline" for older adults who live alone, other forms of technology may also play important roles in older adults' lives. Technology provides home security, access to health care and health information, access to banking from home, and a communications network. The likelihood exists that training of older adults in the use of these helping technologies may facilitate their use and success. Seniors-On-Line (SOL) is a program which provides such training by involving older adults as teachers of classes on computer and Internet use (Irizarry, Downing, & Elford, 1997). The SOL office is staffed 35 hours each week by graduates of previous courses who function as course coordinators. The program consists of eight two-hour classes conducted over a four-week period with opportunities for students to attend additional supervised weekly practice sessions. A 98 percent completion rate has been reported among those who begin the program. Course content includes achievement of a working knowledge of hardware, software, windows operating system, and word processing including tables, spreadsheets, and drawing. It was reported that 70 percent of participants gave "keeping up with modern technology" as their main reason for attending (Irizarry, Downing, & Elford,

1997, p. 42). Reasons given included "keeping an active mind, personal enjoyment, having more in common with younger generations, and acquiring skills for particular tasks" (p. 42). The participants listed the following factors as most helpful in their learning to use computers: program participants in their own age group, freedom to ask questions, individualized help, small classes, and the teachers' communication styles. Also listed as helpful were informal atmosphere, pace of presentation, and teachers in their own age group.

Departing from face-to-face classroom computer training, SeniorNet is reported to be the world's largest trainer of older adults in the use of computer technology (Furlong, 1989). The program began in 1986 at the University of San Francisco, and was designed to ascertain the extent to which telecommunications technology could enhance older adults' lives. Five SeniorNet sites were initially created across the United States, where older adults could learn how to use computers and telecommunications technology. During the early years, the classes were filled as soon as they were announced. The project also created the first online network for seniors and resulted in an online community. SeniorNet provides information on a myriad of topics ranging from health education to legislative initiatives related to older adults. Additionally, the online chat groups provide immediate social networks for those who may be housebound. In addition to health information for seniors, research is cited about the numbers of older adults who use computers, and the type and extent of their use. SeniorNet is another helping technology aimed at facilitating older adults' independence.

Considered together, the helping technologies available to older adults offer at least partial solutions to some of the difficulties encountered when living alone, despite waning functional ability, declining health, and geographic distance from family members. However, these technologies, similar to those used in diagnosis, monitoring, and treatment of illness, cannot function in their designated ways without human interaction. This type of human interaction quite naturally fits within the domain of nursing. Nurses have the ability to provide a caring interface between older adults and the technological inventions needed to maximize their health and independence.

NURSING'S ROLE IN MERGING INVENTIONS EFFECTIVELY

Rapid advancement of helping, diagnostic, monitoring, and treatment technology has placed a new emphasis on the nursing invention of caring. Nurse caring can be the connection between older adults and the technology that may facilitate their health. In light of such concerns as the relationship between anxiety of older adults and computer and ATM technology, nurses have a strong imperative to provide this connection. Nurse caring in the form of empathy, compassion, recognition, and respect for older adults as persons may help to lessen the anxiety that technology seems to engender. This caring also includes teaching about the need, purpose, and function of the technology.

Teaching may be most critical in light of the increased accessibility of health-related information. Because older adults may access information from a dizzying array of sources, there is an ever-increasing demand for nurses to merge their invention—caring—with the information output of technological inventions to facilitate older adults' health. This merging may involve correcting erroneous information, clarifying disturbing or confusing information, as well as doing traditional health teaching.

If nursing fails to fulfill this role, it may be that technological invention will replace nurses as the premier source of health information. Nurses must be aware of the myriad of information sources available to older adults. However, this awareness cannot occur unless nurses ask patients from what sources they usually receive health information, and what information they have about their health. The multiplicity of technological information sources available has made it necessary for nurses to drop the assumption that most health information is received from health care professionals. It is an abdication of the nurse's role to fail to challenge the assumption that information obtained by older adults from the worldwide web and from other sources is reliable. The symbiosis between technology and nursing implies interdependence. In the case of information sources, nurses are essential to interpret, clarify, and correct what older adults learn about their health. In this way, nurses merge caring with technology.

Because of the rapid advancement of technology, and the likelihood that not all segments of older adults will be equally receptive to it in their care or for their own personal use, rapid evolution is needed in merging technology and nurse caring, to be able to address their health care needs. The gap between technological advances used by contemporary nurses and the receptivity of older adults to these technologies may presently be wider than in subsequent cohorts of older adults and nurses. However, nurse caring, by teaching older adult patients about the technologies used in their care, will continue to be critically important as patients struggle to integrate future quantum leaps in technology. Thus, in order to do as Benjamin Franklin suggested, nurses must give freely and generously of their invention caring, so that their older adult patients may enjoy the great advantages of technological inventions through greater independence, health, and effective management of health problems that they encounter.

REFERENCES

Baldi, R. (1997). Training older adults to use the computer: Issues related to the workplace, attitudes and training. *Educational Gerontology, 23*(5), 453–465.

Birdi, K., & Zapf, D. (1997). Age differences in reactions to errors in computer-based work. *Behaviour and Information Technology, 16*(6), 309–319.

Coombs, F. (1994). Engineering technology in rehabilitation of older adults. *Experimental Aging Research, 20*(1), 201–209.

Czaja, S., & Sharit, J. (1998). Age differences in attitudes toward computers. *Journals of Gerontology Series B—Psychological Sciences & Social Sciences, 53B*(5), P329–P340.

Dibner, A. (1990). Personal emergency response systems: Communication technology aids elderly and their families. *Journal of Applied Gerontology, 9*(4), 504–510.

Dyck, J., & Smither, J. A. (1994). Age differences in computer anxiety: The role of computer experience, gender and education. *Journal of Educational Computing Research, 10*(3), 239–248.

Dyck, J., & Smither, J. A. (1996). Older adults' acquisition of word processing: The contribution of cognitive abilities and computer anxiety. *Computers in Human Behavior, 12*(1), 107–119.

Franklin, B. (1966). *The autobiography of Benjamin Franklin.* New York: Washington Square Press.

Furlong, M. (1989). An electronic community for older adults: The SeniorNet Network. *Journal of Communication, 39*(3), 145–153.

Hutchison, D., Eastman, C., & Tirrito, T. (1997). Designing user interfaces for older adults. *Educational Gerontology, 23*(6), 497–513.

Irizarry, C., Downing, A., & Elford, C. (1997). Seniors-On-Line: Introducing older people to technology. *Australasian Physical & Engineering Science in Medicine, 20*(1), 39–43.

Jenkins, R. (2000). *Telemedicine technology: Innovations in home health nursing for congestive heart failure.* Unpublished poster presentation. University of Missouri, Columbia, MO.

Kelley, C., Morrell, R., Park, D., & Mayhorn, C. (1999). Predictors of electronic bulletin board system use in older adults. *Educational Gerontology, 25*(1), 19–35.

Laguna, K., & Babcock, R. (1997). Computer anxiety in young and older adults: Implications for human-computer interactions in older populations. *Computers in Human Behavior, 13*(3), 317–326.

Locsin, L. (1995). Machine technologies and caring in nursing. *Image: Journal of Nursing Scholarship, 27*(3), 201–203.

Marquie, J., Thon, B., & Baracat, B. (1994). Age influence on attitudes of office workers faced with new computer technologies. *Applied Ergonomics, 25*(3), 130–142.

Rogers, W., Cabrera, E., Walker, N., & Gilbert, K. (1996). A survey of automatic teller machine usage across the adult life span. *Human Factors, 38*(1), 156–166.

Ruchlin, S., & Morris, J. (1981). Cost-benefit analysis of an emergency alarm and response system: A case study of a long-term care program. *Health Services Research, 16*(1), 65–80.

SeniorNet. http://www.seniornet.org.

Smither, J. A., & Braun, C. (1994). Technology and older adults: Factors affecting the adoption of automatic teller machines. *Journal of General Psychology, 12*(4), 381–389.

Temple, L., & Gavillet, M. (1990). The development of computer confidence in seniors: An assessment of changes in computer anxiety and computer literacy. *Activities, Adaptation & Aging, 14*(3), 63–76.

Watson, J. (1985). *Nursing: Human science and human caring.* New York: National League for Nursing.

Weil, M., Rosen, L., & Wugalter, S. (1990). The etiology of computerphobia. *Computers in Human Behavior, 6*(4), 361–369.

Chapter 12

Challenging Contemporary Practices in Critical Care Settings

Marian C. Turkel

INTRODUCTION

The critical care environment provides a unique opportunity for nurses to harmonize a seemingly dichotomous practice of technological competency and caring in nursing. Historically, the foci of standards of practice in critical care nursing were proficiency in the area of technology and knowledge about the pathology of disease. Recently, the American Association of Critical Care Nurses (AACN) reconceptualized standards of practice, and the Synergy Model was embraced for critical care nursing practice in the new millennium. In this model of practice, nursing competencies include advocacy, vigilance, engagement, responsiveness, and caring practices (Curley, 1998). Critical care nurses are expected to orchestrate a plan of care integrating these concepts in a highly technological area of nursing practice. Managers of critical care areas need to create environments of caring so nurses have the freedom to engage in caring behaviors in the lived world of practice. The aim of this chapter is to clarify and propose strategies for implementing caring into the contemporary practices of nursing in critical care settings, from the perspective of nurses and nurse managers. The first part of the chapter provides the reader with the theoretical conceptualizations of caring and technology. In the second part of the chapter, challenges to contemporary practices in critical care settings come alive through exemplars and vignettes. Consequently, the reader will note a change in writing style.

NURSING PRACTICE: A PAST GROUNDED IN TECHNOLOGY

In the late 1960s, critical care nursing emerged as a distinct area of nursing practice. The advent of sophisticated monitoring systems and advanced technology meant nurses were capable of more accurate diagnosis and refined treatment of critically ill patients. Standards for critical care nursing practice were developed to articulate the expected competencies of the professional nurse. These standards included proficiency in disease management, proficiency in pathophysiology of disease, and nursing interventions based on the medical model of practice. Another major competency expected of the critical care nurse was the performance of technological skills. These skills included hemodynamic monitoring, EKG interpretation, medication administration, defibrillation, and ventilator management. In 1973, the AACN developed certification examinations to determine and certify expertise of registered nurses practicing in the specialty of critical care (Biel, 1997). These examinations focused on the aforementioned competencies based solely on the clinical judgment facet of critical care nursing practice.

The historical conceptualization of critical care nursing delineated clinical practice dimensions according to a patient's diagnosis and physiological response to a disease. Although nurses may have recognized the value of caring or expressed caring in their practice, caring as a concept of nursing was not reflected in the written standards or competency assessment tools, nor was it expected. From a philosophical point of view, critical care nursing reflected a mechanistic perspective from which the biomedical model of nursing was well served.

CARING IN NURSING

The phenomenon of caring has been identified by many nurse scholars as the essence and core of the practice of nursing (Boykin & Schoenhofer, 1993; Leininger, 1981; Ray, 1994; Watson, 1985, 1988). To Leininger (1981), the most unifying, dominant, and central intellectual and practice focus in nursing is caring. Watson and Leininger used the framework of nursing theory to conceptualize the belief that caring is a central focus for nursing.

In the 1980s, the intensity of discourse on the topic of caring began to increase, in large part due to the influence of Leininger and Watson. The first National Research Conference on Human Care was held in 1978 at the University of Utah (Leininger, 1981). As a result of this conference, varying frameworks for caring were developed, recognized, and published by the scholars in attendance.

Leininger (1981) explicated the idea that caring is the essence of nursing practice and recognized the importance of studying the phenomenon of caring from a theoretical and research perspective. Doing so directed the advancement of the perspective of caring in different cultures and subcultures, enhancing the importance of understanding the meaning of caring for individual groups. By valuing these differing meanings, nursing practice can be more responsive to individual patient requisites. Leininger maintained that differences existed between the essential nature of caring and curing when she claimed that "there can be no curing without caring, but there can be caring without curing" (p. 11). Developing models of practice bearing culture as perspective of care may be necessary in order to advance the understanding of the influences of culture in health care.

Watson (1985) described caring as the "core" of nursing and developed a philosophy and science of caring from a humanistic perspective. Watson's theory examined human science and human care as a framework for nursing practice—defining human caring in nursing as a moral ideal. The nurse carries a caring consciousness in every nursing transaction as an ideal that helps to point the way toward certain human caring actions (Watson, 1990). Transpersonal caring (Watson, 1985) between the nurse and the patient allows the nurse to enter into the world of the patient, wherein the patient consequently enters the nurse's world. In this process, both the patient and nurse move toward the transcendence occurring in a transpersonal caring moment. The human caring process demonstrates respect for the individual humanness of both the nurse and the patient in a transpersonal caring relationship. In a caring transaction, caring is a moral ideal and entails a commitment to a particular end. The end is "the protection, enhancement, and preservation of the person's humanity, which help to restore inner harmony and potential healing" (Watson, 1985, p. 280). To Watson, such an ideal guides the caring actions of nurses as they interact with patients.

Boykin and Schoenhofer (1993) advanced the theory of Nursing As Caring as a framework for practice in the "real world of nursing." In this theory, the nurse enters the world of the nursed with the intention of knowing the other as a caring person. This shared lived experience between nurse and nursed is conceptualized as the nursing situation (Boykin & Schoenhofer, 1993). When nursing practice is approached from the perspective of Nursing As Caring, all persons are known to be caring, living caring in their everyday world.

The currency of Nursing As Caring as a model for transforming practice allows for the contemporary direction of practice issues of health care emphasizing outcomes. Boykin and Schoenhofer (1997) provided descriptions of ways of identifying and understanding outcomes of care through the lens of Nursing As Caring. The traditional language of nursing outcomes is derived from the disciplines of medicine and economics, while Nursing As Caring illuminates caring values as outcomes of nursing practice in the richness and beauty of the nursing situation.

HARMONIC CONVERGENCE OF CARING AND TECHNOLOGY

The seemingly dichotomous nature of caring and technology has been explicated by many nurse scholars (Cooper, 1993; Locsin, 1995, 1998; Ray, 1987; Schoenhofer & Boykin, 1998; Walters, 1995a). Cooper (1993) contends that "nowhere is the paradoxical nature of the relationship between technology, an offshoot of science, and care more evident than in the microculture of an intensive care unit, where the dominance of technology renders many experiences of care invisible or at best obscured" (p. 24). Ray's (1987) germinal research on technology and caring focused on the synthesis of technical nursing competence and humanistic caring in the critical care environment. Ray described the following themes: maturation, technical competence, transpersonal caring, communication, and ethical decision making as components of technological caring—the achievement of caring in critical care nursing.

Walters (1995a) advanced the idea of caring and technology being harmonic forces in the lived world of critical care nursing. The phenomenological approach was used to explore caring in an intensive care unit. The following themes were described: being busy, comforting, focusing, and balancing. These findings enhanced the image of critical care nursing as a harmonic convergence of caring and technology. While Locsin (1995) echoed Walters' idea of harmonizing caring and technology in nursing, Ozbolt (1996) challenged nurses to use the technology to free themselves for caring. Technology is viewed as an enhancement to nursing, rather than an alienation from caring.

Taking a slightly different approach, Locsin (1998) exemplified technological competence as caring in critical care nursing. To Locsin, a nurse who is technologically proficient but does not know the patient fully as a person in the moment is merely a technologist. Technical competencies as expressions of caring are portrayed by critical care nurses who are technologically proficient while responding authentically and intentionally to calls for nursing (Locsin, 1995). "Authenticity and intentionality are demonstrated when the critical care nurse, with all the demands of technologic expertise, accepts the patient fully as a caring person" (Locsin, 1998, p. 54). In the nursing situation, the critical care nurse uses technology to enhance his or her knowledge of the patient as a caring person.

Nursing practice by a critical care nurse is vital in high-technology environments. In this decade, technological advancements continue to dominate technologies of nursing. The health care system has undergone rapid change, and meeting the combined demands of high technology and the profit-driven health care system means that nursing practices must be understood, recognized, and valued as measurable commodities of health care outcomes.

Responding to this demand, Schoenhofer and Boykin (1998) explored outcomes of caring in high-technology environments. In this research study, critical care nurses were found to reaffirm the value of nursing— claiming that "the human component of caring intertwined with the high-tech interventions makes selfless acts of empathy and human sharing possible" (p. 38). This reflection illuminates caring outcomes from a nursing practice that is possible when technology is viewed as an intentional mode of expressing caring (Schoenhofer & Boykin, 1998).

PRACTICE EXEMPLARS: REAFFIRMING CRITICAL CARE NURSING PRACTICE

From a theoretical foundation explicating the harmonious convergence of caring and technology, such a conceptualization needs to be lived in practice. Following are vignettes and situations that make this harmonious coexistence live meaningfully in practice. Intended in the following section is a more personal approach, often using the "first person" as a way to make the presentation of the nursing situations more purposeful and significant, thus illustrating how this theoretical framework can be used to enhance and guide practice.

The Synergy Model: Reconceptualizing Critical Care Nursing

During the past decade, the AACN acknowledged the changing health care environment and sought to develop a new model for practice. The Synergy Model, a reconceptualized model of practice based on the concept that the needs of patients and families drive the competencies of critical care nurses (Biel, 1997), was received as the practice model responsive to contemporary critical care nursing demands. As a framework for certified practice, the following competencies were identified as integral for successful practice: advocacy, caring practices, collaboration, response to diversity, and role of facilitator. Caring practices include, but are not limited to vigilance, engagement, and responsiveness. The Synergy Model is being used as a blueprint for the certification of adult, neonatal, and pediatric critical care nurses. As of July 1, 1999, 80 percent of the examination concept is focused on clinical judgment, and 20 percent on professional caring and ethical practice (AACN, 1999). From a philosophical viewpoint, the Synergy Model reflects a paradigm shift from the mechanistic perspective grounding critical care nursing to a holistic, humanistic perspective of nursing. Using this framework creates a practice of critical care nursing that is challenging while illuminating the art of professional caring.

The Synergy Model clearly articulates the essence of the nurse–patient–family relationship. Within this model, the nurse, the patient, and the patient's family are co-participants. The synergy among all three allows for reciprocal caring interactions and the co-creation of an environment where patient outcomes are optimized. In doing so, critical care nurses are expected to orchestrate a plan of care integrating the concepts of the Synergy Model in high-technology environments. Creating caring environments becomes crucial to nurse managers who are responsible for engaging nurses in the practice of professional caring in critical care arenas.

The Response of Nursing

What would happen if the concepts of being there, authentic presence, knowing patient as person, or holistic caring were also addressed as critical care nursing competencies? The foundation for professional caring is the blending of the humanistic and technical aspects of care. In today's high-technology environments, the critical care nurse needs to focus on "being, knowing, and doing all at once" (Turkel, 1997). This means the nurse needs to integrate caring, knowledge, and skills all at once. Given the current economic constraints, caring in nursing cannot occur in isolation of meeting the physical needs of patients.

While the Synergy Model of nursing in critical care nursing may be the prescribed answer to contemporary critical care nursing, it is important that critical care nurses continue to search for differing approaches to professional practice, allowing the coexistence of caring and technological competency in an increasingly cost-driven health care environment. Doing more with less no longer works; nurses must move outside of the box of contemporary practice to create innovative practice models that explicate cost-effective nursing practice grounded in caring. Challenges such as this can be addressed by remembering the old adage: It takes courage to question the rules, to stretch beyond the comfort zone, and to take risks to change the status quo.

Consider the story of a nurse who is affirming the value of a caring presence in the lived world of practice by allowing family members to remain at the bedside during a cardiac arrest situation or "Code Blue" (Meo, 1998). In this situation, a family member observing the Code Blue team at work realizes firsthand that everything is being done to save the loved one's life. Another nurse reflected on how allowing a family member into a child's room during a Code Blue almost resulted in her being terminated (Meyers, 2000). However, in this situation, the nurse continued to passionately advocate for family presence during resuscitation and invasive procedures. As a result of her perseverance, this practice was ultimately changed, and the hospital now allows family members of the concerned patient to be present during resuscitation, and when invasive procedures are performed.

Many critical care units have open visiting hours to meet the needs of the patients and families. Others allow children and pets to visit as a way of alleviating the anxiety and fear of hospitalization, and to comfort the critically ill patients. Similarly, research studies have affirmed that keeping families in waiting rooms makes them more stressed and anxious (Leske, 1998; Stannard, 1998). In contrast, open visitation hours, family attendance at bedside rounds, and participation in direct care activities foster a trusting relationship between the nurse and the family increasing both patient and family satisfaction (Eagleton & Goldman, 1997; Leske, 1998). Developing a caring relationship between the nurse and the family is imperative in the increasingly competitive health care environment. It was found that what patients and their families remember most at time of discharge is the caring and compassion of the nurse (Eagleton & Goldman, 1997). Patients remember the nurses who took the time to connect with them as a human being with needs and feelings.

Responding as Nursing

Caring practices embraced by the Synergy Model include vigilance, engagement, and responsiveness. Caring practices include not only what nurses do, but also how they do it. Essential to the process of caring is the nurse's recognition of the worth of the patient and the patient's family, and ability to know and care for self (Curley, 1998). The first of these caring practices is vigilance.

Vigilance is defined as alert watchfulness to avoid danger; highly skilled practice, beyond the basics; and nurturing (Burfitt et al., 1993). Critical care nurses express vigilance in practice in many impressive ways. Some examples present these ways as follows:

- Nurses are continuously monitoring the patients' physical conditions while conveying a reassuring presence.
- Nurses are voicing concerns about unsafe care and campaigning to maintain a safe nurse–patient ratio so vigilance is not compromised (Walters, 1995b).
- Nurses have become engaged in advanced practice roles in acute care settings to increase clinical proficiency.
- Nurses are establishing a special connectedness between themselves and families of critically ill patients (Walters, 1995b).
- Nurses are incorporating holistic modalities into practice as a way of nurturing.

Engagement. The unique gift a critical care nurse has to offer to both patients and families is to share self by being truly present with another. Being truly present is an experience of genuinely engaging with another, perhaps for only a moment, perhaps for an extended period of time (Liehr, 1989). To understand "engagement" as a concept of practice in the Synergy Model, the following story is presented.

Probably the one that sticks in my mind more than any is the man that was dying. We had, if you will, a special time together, and that was between 12 and 12:30. And he had made the decision with his wife that he was going to stop everything. He was ready to die. He stopped dialysis. He stopped everything. But our time was 12 to 12:30. I would go in, and I would feed him and we would talk. We'd watch the news and we'd talk about the news. Everybody knew that they would find me in that room from 12 to 12:30. And he said to me, "Today's my day. Today I'm going to meet my maker." And I said, "Are you ready?" He said, "I'm ready." And I said, "Well, you've seen your family. Is there anything else that I can do for you?" And he said, "Yes. One thing." And I said, "What's that?" He said, "I want lasagna." And I said, "Lasagna?" He said, "I want lasagna." So I called the kitchen and said, "Could you fix me up some lasagna?" And they said, "Yes, we can." They brought his lunch in and he had everything he wanted on that tray. And we sat there, and from 12 to 12:30 was our time, and everybody kept coming in. He kept saying, "You're really busy. Do you need to leave?" And I said, "No. Finish your lunch." And he said, "This is so good." I said, "Well, I'm glad." So he kept saying, "They're going to take you from me. They're going to take you from me, they're going to take you from me." He finished his meal and he said, "That was the best meal I've had in years." I said, I'm glad." He said, "Now you go and you take care of all those people out there. And I said, "Okay." And then he started to sing. He sang, "I feel so good right now. I could die right now." And he died right there holding my hand. He died.... I think he knew that he was going to die, ... I'll never forget him. Never in all my life will I ever forget him. Never.... It was the utmost. The utmost. To know that I was a part of his life and his death. (Turkel, 1997, pp. 94–95)

Being truly present for the other is often difficult for nurses to put into words, because it implies engagement and being with the other, rather than doing tasks. The aforementioned story serves as a poignant reminder of the unique gift of being truly present that critical care nurses bring to patients.

Responsiveness requires the nurse to know the patient in order to respond to both physical and emotional needs. Boykin and Schoenhofer (1993) described coming to know the patient as caring person as reflecting the aesthetics of nursing. The phenomenon of knowing the patient also refers to how a nurse understands the patient, grasps the meaning of a situation for the patient, or recognizes the need for a particular intervention (Tanner et al., 1993). Knowing the patient can be conceptualized as knowing the patient as caring person and knowing the patient's pattern of response.

To illustrate this concept, Tanner et al. (1993) asked nurses to share stories of what "knowing the patient" means in the everyday world of practice. The following example illustrates a nurse's description:

It's something, I think, that's hard to describe, but I find with most patients, I feel like I get to know them differently than when they're normal, I'm sure. There is some sense of who this person is. It's when you touch them, or when you say something to them, what happens on their monitors. Or maybe just to see what the effect of what you're doing shows up in what's happening, to the patient, how they look, even when they're paralyzed, just whether their features look a little different, something looks different about them, if they seem to be comfortable when you are there. (p. 275)

The process of knowing the patient shaped the caring activities of the nurse during ventilator weaning and reflected the connection between technology and caring. Responsiveness came alive in the process of knowing the patient, making the Synergy Model more meaningful in nursing patients in critical care settings.

Creating Caring Environments. Nursing administrative practice grounded in caring allows caring and creativity to flourish among the nursing staff. To Cara (1999), staff nurses realized the positive and negative influences of managers on their ability to integrate caring into nursing practice. If nurse managers exhibited more humanistic and caring behaviors, it followed that the nursing staff reflected these in their practice. On the other hand, nurses perceiving an obstructive environment such as a dissonance of values, bureaucracy, abandonment, and oppression create practice behaviors that focus less on a caring practice (Cara, 1999).

Caring Attributes of Nurse Managers. Nursing management is responsible for the way caring is lived and practiced within the organization. Nyberg (1998) encourages nurse managers to "exemplify caring and thus enrich the patient care environment by insisting on the development of an emphasis on caring behaviors throughout the nursing division" (p. 11). According to Nyberg (1998), five attributes enable nurse managers to exhibit caring behaviors: commitment, self-worth, ability to prioritize, openness, and ability to bring out potential. By focusing on the development of these attributes, the nurse manager can be the role model for living caring in the reality of everyday practice.

In today's complex and dynamic environment, nurse managers need to focus on these attributes to be able to work with, through, and to influence staff nurses and other members of the organization. A caring leader acts with integrity by adhering to personal values, principles, and commitments, even when challenged.

Caring for Self. Sister Simone Roach (1987) describes competence as "having the needed skills, judgement and energy required for technical proficiency." However, how many nursing administrators focus on the energy aspect of competence? Are caring-for-self strategies part of management or staff orientation? Is caring for self valued by nursing administration? Considering that high-technology environments are high-stress environments and that critical care nurses are often devastated following a patient's death, it is essential for managers of critical care units to respect and value the concept of caring for self. Following are examples of how nurse managers can use caring-for-self activities in practice:

- Model caring for self by striving for well-being and maintaining a balance between the demands of work and time for self-renewal.
- Start the unit workday with a centering or relaxation experience.
- Allow for mini-relaxation experiences during the course of a 12-hour shift.
- Invite a holistic nurse practitioner to a monthly staff meeting.
- Incorporate caring-for-self activities into the traditional staff development programs.
- Honor the request from a member of the nursing staff to take time off for personal renewal or reflection.

Re-creating Organizational Culture. By transforming the perspective on time management, nurse managers can create a culture that will help nurses and organizations to rediscover their values, their mission, their creativity, and even their productivity. Strategies for re-creating organizational culture include:

- As a hospital organization, dedicate a regular time each month for nurses to contemplate and communicate their visions and goals for the organization.
- Provide a public and private sharing forum, and then as a manager, follow up on the ideas.
- Provide nurses with a "healing room" where they can meditate, rest, or simply reflect on their thoughts. In time, you may begin to see them creatively solving more challenges on their own without intervention from management.
- Set aside time each day for creative/reflective thinking. Post these times in plain sight and encourage all nurses to attend.

Creating a Healing Environment. Nightingale (1859/1969) contended that the role of the nurse was to monitor the environment and make improvements as needed so nature could act to cure the patient. From this perspective, creating a healing environment centers on cleanliness, providing adequate ventilation, keeping the room as quiet as possible, providing a television or a radio, lowering the lights at night, and maintaining patient safety.

Nurse managers and critical care nurses can mutually find ways to facilitate the creation of healing environments. At St. Luke's Episcopal Hospital, advocating innovative design in the critical care environment facilitated the refurbishing of ICU walls with murals of attractive natural landscapes, making the light fixtures look like clouds, and installing piped-in relaxing music (Gray, 1995).

For critical care nurses, environment no longer encompasses only the patient's immediate physical environment. Human beings inhabit a toxic world, where the products and by-products of a technologic society are poisoning our earth and its inhabitants (Schuster & Keegan, 2000). As nursing practitioners who are grounded in caring, awareness of environmental hazards within the health care setting is imperative. Nurses need to increase their knowledge of toxic exposure as they relate to the care of patients in a burgeoning health care industry.

CONCLUDING REMARKS

A delicate balance is at work each time a critical care nurse enters a patient's room. There is a call for nursing that involves the application of knowledge based on complex technology and the intricacies of physiology, and the simultaneous nursing response of caring. Despite the intense focus on technology within the critical care environment, nurses need to reflect on shared meanings as ways of encountering caring in nursing. Nurses are privileged to respond to the call for nursing by offering authentic, intentional, and true caring in the presence of those whom we nurse.

REFERENCES

American Association of Critical Care Nurses (AACN). (1999). *CCRN exam is now based on synergy model.* Aliso Viejo, CA: AACN.

Biel, M. (1997). *Reconceptualizing certified practice: Envisioning critical care practice of the future.* Aliso Viejo, CA: American Association of Critical Care Nurses.

Boykin, A., & Schoenhofer, S. (1993). *Nursing as caring: A model for transforming practice.* New York: National League for Nursing.

Boykin, A., & Schoenhofer, S. (1997). Reframing outcomes: Enhancing personhood. *Advanced Practice Nursing Quarterly, 3,* 60–65.

Burfitt, S., Greiner, D., Miers, L., Kinney, M., & Branyon, M. (1993). Professional nurse caring as perceived by critically ill patients: A phenomenologic study. *American Journal of Critical Care, 2*(6), 489–499.

Cara, C. (1999). Relational caring inquiry: Nurses' perspective on how management can promote a caring practice. *International Journal for Human Caring,* 3(1), 22–30.

Cooper, M. (1993). The intersection of technology and care in the ICU. *Advances in Nursing Science, 15*(3), 23–32.

Curley, M. (1998). Patient-nurse synergy: Optimizing patients' outcomes. *American Journal of Critical Care, 7*(1), 64–72.

Eagleton, B., & Goldman, L. (1997). The quality connection: Satisfaction of patients and their families. *Critical Care Nurse, 17*(6), 76–80, 100.

Gray, B. (1995). What heals: What do nurses do that makes a difference? *Critical Care Nurse Supplement, 15*(3), 3–16.

Leininger, M. (1981). The phenomena of caring: Importance, research questions, and theoretical considerations. In M. Leininger (Ed.), *Caring: An essential human need* (pp. 3–15). Thorofare, NJ: C. B. Slack.

Leske, J. (1998). Interventions to decrease family anxiety. *Critical Care Nurse, 18*(4), 92–95.

Liehr, P. (1989). The core of true presence: A loving center. *Nursing Science Quarterly, 2*(1), 7–8.

Locsin, R. (1995). Machine technologies and caring in nursing. *Image: Journal of Nursing Scholarship, 27*(3), 201–204.

Locsin, R. (1998). Technologic competence as caring in critical care nursing. *Holistic Nursing Practice, 12*(4), 50–56.

Meo, P. (1998, September 8). Til death do we part. *Nursing Spectrum, 8*(18), 7.

Meyers, T. (2000). Why couldn't I have seen him? *American Journal of Nursing, 100*(2), 9–10.

Nightingale, F. (1969). *Notes on nursing: What it is and what it is not.* Philadelphia: Lippincott. Original work published in 1859.

Nyberg, J. (1998). *A caring approach in nursing administration.* Niwot: University of Colorado Press.

Ozbolt, J. (1996). Nursing and technology: A dialectic. *Holistic Nursing Practice, 11*(1), 1–5.

Ray, M. (1987). Technological caring: A new model in critical care. *Dimensions in Cultural Care, 6*(3), 166–173.

Ray, M. (1994). Complex caring dynamics: A unifying model of nursing inquiry. *Theoretic and Applied Chaos in Nursing, 1*(1), 23–32.

Roach, S. (1987). *The human act of caring.* Ottawa: Canadian Hospital Association.

Schoenhofer, S., & Boykin, A. (1998). Value of nursing in high-technology environments. *Holistic Nursing Practice, 12*(4), 31–39.

Schuster, E., & Keegan, L. (2000). *Environment.* In B. Dossey, L. Keegan, & C. Guzzetta (Eds.), *Holistic nursing: A handbook for practice* (3rd ed.) (pp. 249–279). Gaithersburg, MD: Aspen.

Stannard, D. (1998). Families and critical care. *Critical Care Nurse, 18*(4), 86–91.

Tanner, C., Benner, P., Chelsa, C., & Gordon, D. (1993). The phenomenology of knowing the patient. *Image: Journal of Nursing Scholarship, 25*(4), 273–280.

Turkel, M. (1997). *Struggling to find a balance: A grounded theory study of the nurse-patient relationship within an economic context.* Unpublished doctoral diss., University of Miami.

Walters, J. (1995a). Technology and the lifeworld of critical care nursing. *Journal of Advanced Nursing, 22*(2), 338–346.

Walters, J. (1995b). A Heideggerian hermeneutic study of the practice of critical care nurses. *Journal of Advanced Nursing, 21*(3), 492–497.

Watson, J. (1985). *Nursing: Human science and human care*. East Norwalk, CT: Appleton-Century-Crofts.

Watson, J. (1988). New dimensions of human caring theory. *Nursing Science Quarterly, 1*(4), 175–181.

Watson, J. (1990). Transpersonal caring: A transcript view of person, health, and healing. In M. Parker (Ed.), *Nursing theories in practice* (pp. 227–288). New York: National League for Nursing.

Part III

Application Issues: Technology and Caring in Nursing

Chapter 13

Cloning the Clone: Marvel of Technology or Nursing Nightmare?

Jill E. Winland-Brown

INTRODUCTION

Consider the following situations:

- A nurse working in the Emergency Department has just cared for a victim of a motorcycle accident who didn't "make it." His wife rushes in, and demands that the nurse obtain a sperm sample because she has been trying to have a baby with her husband and knows that this is her last chance. She wants a child to be a reminder of their love shared. What would you do?
- A young family just had their only child diagnosed with a rare neurological disease. Their only hope is to have another baby and donate its healthy stem cells to their child, hopefully to correct the problem. What would you do?
- The child of an elderly couple drowns. For 20 years they have tried to have a baby and rejoiced when their son was born. Now the child is dead and they have no one to carry on their legacy. They want to clone the baby so they can continue caring for the child for whom they had waited so long. What would you do?

Years ago, these scenarios may have sounded like science fiction. Today, the first two scenarios have already happened and the third is very feasible. These complex situations directly challenge nursing and caring as the essence of nursing. Who is the patient in each of these situations? Who are nurses to serve and protect? The parents? The child? Assisted reproductive technologies (ART) and other technologies today demand that nurses respond with care. Nurses must be prepared and respond to situations such as these by being proactive, rather than reactive. This chapter offers an overview of these complex, "on the edge" biogenic technologies that face nurses in contemporary health care.

THE BENEFITS OF RESEARCH

Research produces many new innovative and useful ideas. Without research, society would not have been able to receive the benefits that exist today in high technology. Examples from history illustrate how the birth of an idea can result in significant contributions from which we all benefit. Through research, scientists aim for great possibilities through many trials and errors. Thomas Edison exemplified determination when he made 10,000 attempts to invent the lightbulb. He claimed he did not have 10,000 failures, but just 10,000 times when the lightbulb did not work. Each attempt gave him more insight toward the next and finally successful attempt. Today, because of Einstein's tenacity, the world relies on a technology which 200 years ago was thought to be impossible.

Twenty-five years ago artificial insemination was seen as so abhorrent that it was even banned for use in cattle. Today, the public acceptance of test-tube babies demonstrates how quickly new technology can become mainstream when it pulls on the heartstrings of those individuals desiring a healthy child (Fielding, 1997). Through the use of assisted reproductive technology (ART), Baby Louise, the first "test-tube baby," was born almost 25 years ago. What used to be called a test-tube baby is now commonly referred to as in-vitro fertilization (IVF), where the oocytes first are fertilized in a laboratory test tube and the resulting embryos are then implanted in a woman's uterus. Over the years ARTs have become commonplace. In 1990, it became a criminal offense to keep an embryo alive for longer than two weeks after fertilization, with a penalty of up to 10 years in prison (Warnock, 1998). Today, vigorous debates take place in courts of law over who has the right to frozen embryos when couples who have together donated the eggs and sperm divorce. Yet the basic premise of ART, that of assisting infertile couples to propagate, allows many people great moments of joy because researchers were given a chance to explore the possibilities of a new frontier.

THE STATE OF CLONING TECHNOLOGY

When we think of cloning, a futuristic society may come to mind in which individuals clone themselves to increase their productivity or to be in two places at once. Michael Keaton portrays such a scenario in the movie *Multiplicity*. While this movie is fiction, it is not unrealistic in this era of high technology.

The first successful cloning technique in vertebrate animals occurred with frogs in 1952 (NBAC, 1998a), but most Americans first started to think about cloning when the media focused attention on a sheep named "Dolly," the first cloned mammal. Dolly was "born" in 1996 when Scottish scientist Ian Wilmut transferred the nucleus of a somatic cell from an adult sheep into an egg from which the nucleus had been removed. This technique had never before been successful. The National Bioethics Advisory Committee (NBAC) formed by President Clinton called this new technology "somatic cell nuclear transfer" (SCNT). Research origins of this cloning technique can be found as far back as 40 years ago (Childress, 1997).

Cloning involves creating a genetic copy or replica (Robertson, 1994). When considering the human implications of cloning, it is necessary to distinguish between cloning by embryo splitting and cloning by nuclear replacement. Nuclear replacement may be distinguished as a means of cloning or as a means of therapeutic utilization. Cloning by embryo splitting, however, involves division of a single embryo, where the divided nuclear genes and some of the mitochondrial genes are an identical "match." Nuclear transfer technology allows selection of nucleus donor cells that express the desired transplanted gene. Companies use this same technique to produce "transgenic" cows that produce albumin for treating persons who have suffered large blood losses. Transgenic cattle also produce the human blood proteins fibrinogen, factor IX, and factor VIII in their milk, which can be used to treat individuals with bleeding disorders. Transgenic pigs are produced to supply needed organs for transplantation.

The Human Genome Project is a $3 billion federal effort expected to be completed in 2003 (Cochran, 1999). Its effort is aimed at gathering scientific information about the human genome with the objective being to locate, identify, and sequence the 100,000 genes on the 46 human chromosomes, and create a blueprint for every trait, disease, and perhaps behavior. The ultimate goal is to produce a map identifying the location of all genes in the human genome and determine the chemical sequence of human deoxyribonucleic acid (DNA). After the human genome is sequenced, drugs will be developed to neutralize the genetic codes of infectious agents such as the human immunodeficiency virus (HIV), tuberculosis (TB), and hepatitis. These genomic scientists claim that many diseases may be helped by cloning; for example, the reversal of heart attacks. If healthy heart cells can be cloned, then injected into the necrotic area of the heart, damage may be reversed. The same procedure may potentially be used for damaged islet cells in the pancreas. Countless other possibilities exist for such a technology, although the actual idea of human cloning seems frightening to many individuals who have not explored all the possibilities, such as the three scenarios described in the beginning of this chapter.

BENEFITS FROM CLONING

The results of genetic testing help clarify, diagnose, and direct patients toward appropriate treatments. At the same time, genetic testing information helps parents avoid giving birth to children with devastating health and physical conditions. An added benefit of genetic testing is identifying at-risk patients who are prone to a preventable disease (Cochran, 1999). The goal in the future is not to *treat* diseases but to *prevent* diseases, since genetic susceptibility of individuals to a number of disorders can be predetermined. Possibilities exist for defective DNA to be replaced through gene therapy.

The benefits of cloning animals have already been realized. A commercial institution in the United States is successfully genetically "engineering" goats to produce a human protein to affect blood clotting. Combining multiple genetic technologies, these goats are then cloned to continue the beneficial effects across generations.

Other companies are growing embryos for stem cells to treat a multitude of chronic ailments, such as Parkinson's disease and diabetes. Ten thousand genetic disorders have been identified. The possibility exists that in the future, diseases such as Parkinson's and diabetes may become diseases or disorders of past generations. Some of the most marketable genes to be developed are those that can manipulate cancer cells, as well as those that may affect obesity and baldness (Belkin, 1998).

Cloning is a method of asexual reproduction. A woman may donate her own DNA, her own unfertilized egg, and her uterus, and create a baby in her own likeness without male involvement. Some may not consider this a benefit, but surely the possibility must be considered (Newman, 1997). Technically, the clone would have no biological parents. The "mother" did not *just* donate her egg, and the "father" does not exist. Whom shall the baby call its parents? Within what social context will the clone be raised? The clone is now reduced to being a commercial product. The calls for nursing in a situation such as this are mind-boggling.

The human imagination can elicit a multitude of potential benefits from cloning, from eliminating devastating diseases to creating humans who are more aesthetically pleasing, with specific physical (blond hair, blue eyes) and creative (musical or athletic ability) attributes. When cloning is mentioned, the possibility of cloning individuals of great talent or genius is usually the first thought that comes to mind. Imagine the implications of cloning a Mozart or an Einstein! The question remains: Is this a benefit, or are we opening "Pandora's box?"

QUESTIONS

While the benefits of cloned animals are presently being enjoyed, the assumption cannot be made that the benefit of cloning of human beings will be of such magnitude as to override the ethical issues that are being presented, which center around the concept of diminished respect for human life. While genetic technology creates new and unique arguments, an analogy can be made with an illustration often cited when new, frightening technologies arise. When airplanes were invented, many claimed that "If God had meant us to fly—he would have given us wings." Yet, the response to this argument is that God gave us the intelligence and creativity to develop our own wings, so we could fly. Within this symbolic argument may be seen the same challenges and conflicts that each new scientific technology creates, such as the technologies of nuclear power and in-vitro fertilization.

In-vitro or test-tube fertilization, while initially causing great socioreligious arguments, did not prevent people from turning to this technology to satisfy their need for children. The primary premise is not the idea of creating or destroying life, but the right of people to use technology that satisfies their needs. This is the inherent argument. Whose right is it, ultimately, to use guns, smoke a carcinogenic product, employ nuclear weapons, assist in one's suicide, or have an abortion?

One common denominator is the need for each individual to achieve his or her personal objectives, whether in desiring to create life, as in the potential of human cloning, or in destroying life, as in abortions. Thus, we come to a primary issue, which is the extent of personal freedom in utilizing the accomplishments of the scientific community. When scientists create technology that people want and can afford to acquire, there will be great difficulty in preventing such acquisition in a democratic society (Executive Summary, 1997; Harris, 1997). This does not support the assumption that the desires of people cannot be denied, for today, people who wish to die are often made to suffer a slow death because as unwanted medical technology keeps them alive. However, when the needs of people and the availability of technology concur, then the ethical arguments of religious and political leaders, as well as social scientists, usually have little effect. Harris (1997) refers to this as procreative autonomy.

ABUSES OF HUMAN CLONING

The somatic cell nuclear transfer technique could easily be used to create children. This raises various complex, ethical issues such as individuality, family integrity, and the possibility of children being treated as objects. With the blurring of family boundaries, where do the fundamental responsibilities rest, especially in regard to intergenerational relationships? According to Carey (1998), cloning is not just an infertility treatment; it is a quantum leap from in-vitro fertilization.

Historically, whenever a procedure or behavior is banned, it is driven underground where unsafe, unregulated, and exploitative misuses may be employed (Carey, 1998). Similar possibilities exist with regard to cloning. Certainly, if one had a choice out of a number of healthy cells to be cloned, and one could predetermine sex or physical characteristics, many persons would choose to clone an athlete such as Michael Jordan or a scientist such as Einstein. Others who could afford the technology may choose to clone a powerful, manipulative person, such as Hitler, thus promulgating more individuals of this kind. While the first situation may be acceptable to some, the second probably would not. A unique human being may cease to exist in the future. Even the term "individual" might become a rarity. Human cloning could eventually be used for commercial purposes, for financial gain (Brock, 1998). Potential parents desiring a blue-eyed, blond-haired baby could order their child from a catalog.

What will happen when patents are allowed on gene fragments? Can there be property rights to individuals? Is life a human invention that can be patented, or is human life a creation of God? Society must answer these questions before technology advances any further. National ethics organizations such as the NBAC, the Kennedy Institute of Ethics at Georgetown University; and/or the Hastings Center, Institute of Society, Ethics and the Life Sciences were created to address issues such as these (see the list at the end of the chapter for ethics organizations).

THE STAKEHOLDERS

In such circumstances, before ethical issues are debated, the first step is to decide who should be involved in the argument. Included in this discussion are all those who have a stake or vested interest in the outcome.

Parents now have the right to have or not to have children, or to decide when to have children. Society and government do not become involved legally in family matters as long as the parents are productive members of society and can provide a stable, loving environment for their children. Should this procreative right of parents be abrogated if the parents decide to clone one of their children and produce an identical sibling with several years' difference in ages? Parents are used to privacy in family matters. If the technology exists, shouldn't parents be entitled to utilize it?

Religious groups historically have been influential in slowing the concepts of technological advancement. There is no single "religious" view on human cloning, and religious perspectives differ. Some religious leaders believe that cloning humans to create children may be justified under some circumstances, while others contend that cloning violates fundamental moral tenets such as human dignity. Most argue for regulation due to potential abuses of the technology (NBAC, 1998b). Public outcry influences lawmakers to the extent that future progress may be impeded.

Scientists who create technology want the recognition of their discoveries (Wilkie & Graham, 1998). Scientists need the freedom to work on developing further discoveries that at first seem alarming, but will eventually provide the groundwork for new technologies to help humankind. This is the impetus that must be protected and preserved in order for new technology to be uncovered. Discoveries such as those which may ameliorate suffering or cure disease are waiting to be harvested, and like any new seedling, need only time and attentiveness to be cultivated (NBAC, 1998a). Yet, many scientists are wary of technology, as it is a quantum leap from cloning frogs in 1952 to cloning humans in the near future (Callahan, 1998).

Lawmakers are stakeholders, as citizens expect them to uphold current standards to protect individual rights. Because of the media attention focused on Dolly, a cloned sheep, the NBAC enacted a five-year legal ban on federally funded research in the area of human cloning. Because the NBAC has jurisdiction only over federally funded projects, this ban is ineffective in cloning research taking place in the private sector (Executive Summary, 1997).

Persons in *industry* and commercial ventures are stakeholders, as they will potentially profit from the publicity and technology. Patents may be sold for pharmaceutical products that are developed with cloning technology, and human cloning laboratories may be operated for profit.

The *media* are able to influence public opinion by presenting views stressing one side of an issue. It takes an astute reader to determine fact from fiction, and truth from hearsay. The press has a lot of power without responsibility (Wilkie & Graham, 1998). One article about Dolly refers to the sheep as a "landmark in biological research," and further states that "cloning is also likely to cause harm" (Wilkie & Graham, 1998, p. 52). The perspective of an article can positively or negatively influence people, even if they originally had opinions leaning in the opposite direction.

In 1997, a movie was produced, entitled *Gattaca*, about a futuristic society where genetically engineered persons were first-class citizens while others, the product of sexual procreation, occupied menial positions. To promote the movie, an advertisement appeared in the media asking persons who wanted designer babies with a "shopping list" of traits to call 1–888–4-BEST-DNA. When individuals called, they received no response. The advertisement was simply a ploy to generate interest in the movie (Ackerman, 1999). Persons responding to this ad were willing to take the first steps in exploring a genetically altered future.

The cloned beings, as the ultimate stakeholders, may possess mixed feelings about the circumstances of their origination or the reason for their existence, as is the case of abortions not being carried out by mothers. They may feel glad they exist, but also be resentful of the person from whom they were cloned. These individuals may feel that they were not the "original," or feel like an "imitation" or a "copy." They may also feel like second-class citizens even while finding value in their existence. Indeed, society may form a "caste-like" society, as the individuals who are cloned are reduced to feeling like a product and to being treated accordingly. Research on identical twins has shown that each twin is constantly compared with the other (Holm, 1998). Imagine the life of a clone that is an exact replica? Living life in the shadow of another "diminishes the clone's possibility of living a life that is in a full sense of that word his or her life" (Holm, 1998, p. 162).

THE ETHICS INVOLVED

The study of ethics is continually racing to keep up with scientific research and technology. The ethics surrounding cloning issues are complex and evolving. Three main ethical principles of autonomy, beneficence, and justice are discussed in relation to cloning.

Autonomy implies self-determination and self-directness. But does personal autonomy allow an individual the right to "self-replicate?" Do humans have a right to their own genetic identity? Human beings should at least have the right to control their own reproductive destiny, as long as no one else is harmed (Harris, 1997). Do persons have the right to control their own bodies—a commitment to individual liberty? "Yes," say infertile heterosexual couples, gay couples, and several single persons paying $200,000 to a cloning company (Carey, 1998). If individuals have the right to donate an organ or tissue, can parents delegate this authority to minors? If an individual does not yet exist, and cloning techniques to produce that child were utilized for the sole purpose of using the resultant tissues or organs, could there be a "wrongful life" suit? (Fitzgerald, 1998).

Nurses have always upheld informed consent as a major component of autonomy. With regard to stem cells, or cloning a child, who ethically should give informed consent? Should the parent who is benefiting from the result? Nurses will be faced with this issue in the near future and must be able to respond. The Center for Ethics and Human Rights of the American Nurses Association customarily takes a stand on issues such as these and publishes a position paper that will assist in guiding practicing nurses who are confronted by these issues.

Yet, autonomy in the realm of biogenic technology in the twenty-first century mandates that the collective whole (society) be considered, as well as individuals. Since the gene pool is the joint property of society and not owned by any one person, when the gene pool is manipulated, society must be in agreement (Anderson, 1999).

Beneficence. A major benefit of cloning is that there is no rejection factor.

The human physiological response to reject foreign bodies or substances does not activate in response to an individual's own DNA. When weighing the pros and cons of organ donation, this fact must be considered true beneficence. There would be a significant impact on health care with regard to the cost saved for anti-rejection drugs, as well as significantly longer lives for many individuals.

Society has come to accept the benefits of in-vitro fertilization (IVF) for infertile couples. Some persons feel that cloning human embryos poses no greater harm to embryos than other IVF techniques. Because of fewer risks and more benefits, these same persons state that cloning should be considered no different from IVF (Robertson, 1994).

Justice. The principle of justice mandates fairness for all, particularly for the most vulnerable in society. Are persons with no health insurance or members of Health Maintenance Organizations (HMOs) considered more vulnerable than others in the population? Will they be able to benefit from high-tech advances in medical science? Conversely, will HMOs use the same genetic information to screen out beneficiaries who have been shown to have genetically related diseases on their records? Will insurance companies deny individuals insurance on the basis of a pre-existing genetic susceptibility? If technology cannot be prohibited, it must at least be regulated. It will never be a poor man's campaign (O'Connor, 1997). Will the ability to access technology be regarded in the future as entitlement or as a right requiring public subsidy?

PANDORA'S BOX OF ETHICAL QUESTIONS

Researchers of eugenics, the study of hereditary improvements, suggest that many Americans want a blond, blue-eyed child (Ackerman, 1999; Brock, 1998). Yet, these same individuals who possess blond, blue-eyed traits are more prone to skin cancer. Every genetic trait has an effect on every other. Recessive traits that are essential for evolutionary functions are present in every gene pool, and many of them have not yet been discovered (Ackerman, 1999). Is society prepared to open Pandora's box?

Society must consider and decide what is an acceptable limit of genetic intervention. Most persons will agree that an acceptable intervention is fighting cancer; fewer probably will agree that genetic intervention might be acceptable for correcting a violent behavior gene. A "slippery slope" argument exists, however, when consideration is given to augmenting traits such as musical or athletic ability (Cochran, 1999). Employing cloning to reproduce human life implies that people are replaceable and are not unique beings. Cloning to replace an individual who has died, for example, has many hidden implications for both parents and for the one who is cloned. The cloned individual may feel that he/she is a "replacement," and the parents may state that if the first child had not died, they would not have cloned him/her. The child needs to be protected from the "lifelong, unpredictable and potentially troubling consequences of cloning" (Newman, 1997, p. 530). Possibilities inherent in the discovery of new technologies do not produce alarm; instead, fear arises in considering where these technologies will be put to use.

CONCLUDING STATEMENTS

When women give birth, they can usually describe, accurately and vividly, the pain involved. An analogy may be made with an oyster, which from the irritation of a painful grain of sand produces a beautiful pearl. The beauty of a new child is like the pearl after the pain. But is the pain comparable if the woman is unable to conceive her own child? If there were a means by which she could conceive a child, and this means was denied her, how then would her pain be measured?

Bioengineers are actively working on reshaping those challenges and presenting new options, not only concerning the ability of a woman to give birth to a new child, but concerning the ability to produce a healthy child devoid of inherent disease and malformations. This is one of many promising alternatives that biogenetic progress holds for the future. "Cloning is not just a Xerox machine for our genes. It's a window into our soul as well"(Carey, 1998). Society still debates over whether life begins at conception. The link between stem cell research and human cloning poses additional new questions. Stem cell research requires that human embryos be 5 to 10 days old. However, a new definition of life generates questions as to whether or not an embryo should be regarded as a person until it is at least 14 days old, when the first evidence of a nervous system appears (*Palm Beach Post*, 1999). The case may be made that, if there is a need and people can afford the technology, and the technology is satisfying their needs while having no negative effect on anyone else, then cloning should be admissible and accepted.

Health care professionals need to consider these issues before being confronted with them. One solution might be to have the American Nurses Association (ANA) survey members and arrive at a collective decision regarding the professional association's stand on the ethical issues of cloning.

The technology to successfully clone human beings may be available in the near future, and may be created whether or not individuals or society take a stand on the issue. So, while cloning may be a marvel of technology, the issues presented here may make it a nursing nightmare. The three scenarios cited at the beginning of this chapter will begin to occur with increasing frequency. Women whose husbands are dying or dead will insist on obtaining sperm to self-impregnate. Women will conceive in order to use the newborn child's stem cells to correct an existing child's disorder or disease. Families will clone children who have died. Fiction will become fact, and nurses will be faced with these issues in the future. At a time when cultural diversity is celebrated, genetic diversity will be reduced. Does this paradox make sense? Nurses committed to care must address these issues of wholeness and uniqueness when genetic identity is in question.

Where to Go for Further Information on Ethics and Cloning Issues

- American Nurses Association Center for Ethics and Human Rights, 600 Maryland Avenue, SW, STE 100 West, Washington, DC 20024–2571, (202) 651–7000. Their quarterly ethics publication is the *Communique*. www.ana.org; also www.nursingworld.org/index.htm
- *Hastings Center Report*. Published bimonthly by the Hastings Center, Garrison, New York, 10524–5555, (914) 424–4040, www.thehastingscenter.org
- *Hospital Ethics*. Published bimonthly by the American Hospital Association, 840 North Lake Shore Dr., Chicago, Illinois 60611.
- *Issues: A Critical Examination of Contemporary Ethical Issues in Health Care*. Published monthly by the SSM Health Care System, 477 N. Lindbergh Blvd., St. Louis, MO 63141.
- *The Journal of Clinical Ethics*. Published quarterly by University Publishing Group, 107 East Church Street, Frederick, MD 21701.
- *Kennedy Institute of Ethics Journal*. Published quarterly by Johns Hopkins University Press, 701 West 40th Street, STE 275, Baltimore, Maryland 21211. In addition, the BIOETHICSLINE database (BIOETHICS) is produced at the Kennedy Institute of Ethics at Georgetown University, and is made available online through the National Library of Medicine's MEDLARS system. BIOETHICS citations appear in print form in the annual *Bibliography of Bioethics*. http://adminweb.goergetown.edu/kennedy
- *Medical Ethics Advisor*. A paper published monthly by American Health Consultant Inc., 3525 Piedmont Road, N.E., Building Six, STE 400, Atlanta, GA 30305.
- *The Journal of Medical Humanities*. Published quarterly by Human Sciences Press, 233 Spring Street, New York, N.Y. 10013.
- *Nursing Ethics: An International Journal for Health Care Professionals*. Published quarterly by Edward Arnold, 338 Euston Road, London NWI 3BH, United Kingdom.

REFERENCES

Ackerman, T. (1999, July 11). Genetic scientists walk ethical tightrope. *Sun Sentinel, South Florida* IG, 3G.

Anderson, F. (1999, July 11). Quoted from Ackerman, T. Genetic scientists walk ethical tightrope. *Sun Sentinel, South Florida*, 1G.

Belkin, L. (1998, August 23). Splice Einstein and Sammy Glick: Add a little Magellan. *The New York Times Magazine*, 26–31, 56–61.

Brock, D. W. (1998). Cloning human beings: An assessment of the ethical issues pro and con. In M. C. Nussbaum & C. R. Sunstein (Eds.), *Facts and fantasies about human cloning*. New York: W. W. Norton.

Callahan, D. (1998). Cloning: Then and now. *Cambridge Quarterly of Healthcare Ethics, 7*(2), 141–144.

Carey, J. (1998, August 10). Commentary: Human clones: It's decision time. *Business Week*.

Childress, J. F. (1997). The challenges of public ethics: Reflection on NBAC's Report. *Hastings Center Report, 27*(5), 9–11.

Cloning human beings: Responding to the National Bioethics Advisory Commission's report. (1997). *Hastings Center Report, 27*(5), 6.

Cochran, J. (1999). Genetic code. *Miami Magazine, 6*(2), 16–21.

Executive Summary. (1997). *From Cloning Human Beings: The Report and Recommendations of the National Bioethics Advisory Commission* (Rockland, MD, June), in *Hastings Center Report, 27*(5), 7–9.

Fielding, E. W. (1997). Fear of cloning. *The Human Life Review, 23*(2), 15–22.

Fitzgerald, K. T. (1998). Proposals for human cloning: A review and ethical evaluation. In J. F. Monagle & D. C. Thomasma, (Eds.), *Health Care Ethics— Critical Issues for the 21st Century* (ch. 1). Gaithersburg, MD: Aspen Publishers.

Harris, J. (1997). Goodbye Dolly? The ethics of human cloning. *Journal of Medical Ethics, 23*(6), 353–360.

Holm, S. (1998). A life in the shadow: One reason why we should not clone humans. *Cambridge Quarterly of Healthcare Ethics, 7*(2), 160–162.

National Biothetics Advisory Committee. (NBAC). (1998a). Ethical aspects of cloning techniques: Opinion of the group of advisers on the ethical implications of biotechnology of the European Commission. *Cambridge Quarterly of Healthcare Ethics, 7*(2), 187–193.

National Bioethics Advisory Committee (NBAC). (1998b). Religious perspectives and human cloning: An historical overview. In M. C. Nussbaum & C. R. Sunstein, *Clones and clones: Facts and fantasies about human cloning*. New York: W. W. Norton.

Newman, S. A. (1997). Human cloning and the family: Reflections on cloning existing children. *New York Law School Journal of Human Rights 13*(3), 523–530.

O'Connor, C. (1997). Human cloning: Efficiency vs. ethics. *Origins, 26*(42), 681–684.

Robertson, J. A. (1994). The question of human cloning. *Hastings Center Report, 2*(24), 6–14.

Scientists try to clone human embryos. (1999, June 14). *Palm Beach Post*, 2.

Warnock, M. (1998). The regulation of technology. *Cambridge Quarterly of Healthcare Ethics, 7*(2), 173–175.

Wilkie, T., & Graham, E. (1998). Power without responsibility: Media portrayals of Dolly and science. *Cambridge Quarterly of Healthcare Ethics, 7*(2), 150–159.

Chapter 14

Technology in a Climate of Restructuring: Contradictions for Nursing

Eileen Willis and Karen Parish

INTRODUCTION: SETTING THE SCENE

The setting for this study is a government-funded, 250-bed Extended Care and Rehabilitation facility, which we have called Belair Services, in a capital city in Australia. This organization provides services for adults with a range of disabilities such as an acquired brain injury or degenerative neurological diseases. The clients within this service are highly dependent and have significant manual-handling needs. In 1995, a review of lifting and positioning practices demonstrated that the use of hydraulic lifters and beds with only manual "high/low" adjustments and no other capacity meant that considerable time was being spent on these activities. There was also a relatively high incidence of manual-handling injuries for nurses, and a view that clients felt vulnerable and afraid during lifts. This led nursing management to argue for the replacement of all existing lifters with electronic lifters, and approximately 75 percent of existing beds with electronic, fully adjustable beds. These costly technologies were introduced with the view that they would be of advantage to both clients and nurses, eventually becoming cost-neutral, allowing the organization to make the necessary, government-imposed budgetary savings.

As a result of the new electronic beds and lifters resident-handling injuries for nurses decreased from 47 injuries in 1995/1996 to 26 in 1997/1998. More importantly, residents reported that the electronic lifters were "smoother," with the adjustable beds providing more comfortable positioning than bolsters and pillows. The increased satisfaction of clients in relation to autonomy and personal feelings of safety was also significant, as was the reduction in client anxiety during lifts. The time savings to nursing hours were also significant, with the new lifts reducing the number of nursing hours needed for a shift, enabling management to meet the staff reduction target.

The above report on the impact of highly expensive, yet effective machinery illustrates the contemporary relationship between technology and its promise of liberating humans from the drudgery of work, suffering, and pain. In the case study, the gains to patient comfort are obvious. However, the full impact of this technology on nursing work and morale is only hinted at. It is noted that while the safety of nursing work was enhanced, the overall nursing work force was decreased. Furthermore, nursing management implemented this change. This chapter explores the possible contradictions between technology that benefits clients introduced within the framework of restructuring and cost-cutting, and the impact this technology has on nurses' labor.

The chapter is divided into two sections. In the first section, we outline the contribution of neo-Marxist theory on work and the labor process as the expression of human creativity, bringing to this discussion the unique position that technology, science, and bureaucracy are accorded, as well as the problem of alienation that arises under capitalist social relations. This enables us to ask broadly based, sociological and structural questions about the positions of staff nurses and nurse managers, in relation to the simplest or most sophisticated technologies, and bureaucratic and managerial decision making. The connecting theme is in the second section, where we provide further examples from Belair Services that describe the introduction of technical innovations accompanied by workplace restructuring. A core concept in our paper is that technological benefits contribute to patient comfort and to the need management has to improve efficiency through either cost-cutting or increasing profits. It is this that makes the nurses' relationship to technology problematic. However, it is not only the nurse at the bedside who experiences this contradiction in his or her caring work, but also nurse managers. Their dilemma is one where they must weigh implications for some nurses against other nurses, as well as for nurses against patients.

CRITICAL THEORY: NURSING, TECHNOLOGY, AND CARE

Marxist Theory of Labor and Technology

Within the sociological literature, technology is understood in broad terms. It is not reduced to machinery or tools, but includes both the techniques of production as well as the way workers, including professionals, are organized in a factory, office, or hospital (Abercrombie, Hill,

& Turner, 1984). Technology is also seen to arise out of human interaction with nature. As will become evident, separating technologies as tools and machinery produced by humans (as they act upon the material world) from the organizational and bureaucratic processes of production of care itself is a difficult task. The two are inextricably linked. Further, to assume that nursing was ever without technology is naive. The bedpan, the cup, and the pillow are technologies, just as is the latest therapy for women with breast cancer or the most recent, computerized tomographic scanner on the market. This points to the idea of evolution embedded in technology. Technology impinges on the very labor or caring process itself, so that it is possible to suggest that the nature of nursing as labor can be transformed.

As medical technologies change, nurses are forced into an ongoing dialectic with the tools of curing and care in their work. Taking a patient's temperature using your own watch given to you on graduation is a simple act of care between nurse and nursed. Attending a meeting where the hospital decides whether to purchase state-of-the-art cardiac monitoring equipment that comes complete with training sessions, morning teas, gifts, ongoing maintenance backup, and network links with other technologies is a complex act involving struggles over budget shortfalls with other units in the institution, staffing numbers and hours, shareholder profits and the pace of work, as well as new ways of nursing and interacting with those in one's care. Technology impinges on the very labor (caring) process itself, so that it is possible to suggest that the nature of nursing as labor can be transformed. This is certainly the experience of nurse managers.

Work, whether it be in the fields, the factory, or in the clinic, occurs in a context that is marked by the forces and means of production and the relations of production (Cheek et al., 1996). The forces of production include human science and technology; the means are the tools and machinery used in production, while the social relations refer to the way that work is organized. Social life in the workplace is a reflection of the technology of the time and the way that work is organized. While it is easy to fall into economic determinism with Marxist analysis, this was not the original intention. For Marx, work was fundamental to humans. It was that which made us human, since it involved providing for our material needs. The way this work (or creative activity) was organized between groups of workers constituted the social relations. The technology was an expression of human creative work and constituted the outward manifestation of our creativity. Waters and Crook (1993) note, "The objects which human beings produce are part of human nature because they are the form of its expression. To separate people from the things which they produce and from the processes by which they are produced is to deny human nature" (p. 423). This separation is what Marx meant by alienation. Comforting and curing technologies, such as analgesics, are a reflection of human creativity at work and presumably are embraced for this very reason. Such technologies offer nurses the potential for liberation from the drudgery of work, and patients freedom from the oppression of pain.

Technology, however, is problematic within social relations of alienation and exploitation. Such problematic areas are found in the social relations of production or work. The (labor) process of caring that confronts most nurses is one where they are waged in the service of either private hospital boards, third-party insurers, HMOs, or the state. While individual nurses may rise to managerial positions and become part of internal decision making, with all its contradictions, they remain essentially employees. Their relationship to the technology is contradictory. Technology is not just a reflection and extension of the nurse's creative and caring work; it is also a commodity. Technology is also used by the nurse in the interests of profit or cost containment, albeit at times unconsciously. For the nurse, this is a relationship of alienation and an example of the degradation of work (Braverman, 1974). Ideas about the conception and execution of work are separated, with management and owners making decisions about what is to be done, while nurses perform the tasks. Caring tasks are performed using tools and machinery over which most nurses have little control, or ownership. Nurses still produce (care), but this is appropriated by the owner of the means of production (Cheek et al., 1996). Medical technologies used in the production of care are also commodity-producing, with the nurses' surplus labor (efficiencies) producing profit or cost containment.

CARING, TECHNOLOGY, RESTRUCTURING, AND LABOR

Any discussion of the impact of medical technology on the way that nurses perform their caring work cannot avoid examining the massive restructuring that has occurred in the health care systems of a number of countries. Within the Western bloc, reorganization and restructuring have been achieved in the British, North American, Scandinavian, Australian, and New Zealand health care systems since the 1990s (Hsiao, 1992). These reforms have been motivated partly by the high cost of maintaining the welfare state, which in turn has been driven by the increasing cost of health care, but also by radical shifts in international labor markets, deregulation, and globalization, and shifts from collectivist to individualist ideologies. Technology, including medical technology, has played a major role in this restructuring, impacting on the labor processes of workers, including the caring work of nurses. These technologies have become essential tools in the reorganization of work, partly because they promise time-based cost savings or extend the life and comfort of patients. Within the industrial relations literature, the impact of these reforms on the labor processes of workers is referred to as a shift from neo- to post-Fordist forms of management, or flexible specialization (Mathews, 1992). The term "Fordism" has its origins in the pioneering work of the American Harry Braverman (1974), who argued that monopoly capitalism differed from early capitalism in the way work was controlled. Drawing on the ideas of Frederick Winslow Taylor, the American inventor of "scientific management," and Henry Ford, who introduced the conveyor belt into his car factory, Braverman's argument is twofold. Braverman suggests that with Taylorism, management began to use the social sciences to control workers so that a split developed between the execution of the task, which was done by the worker, and the idea of the task, which was controlled by management. This analysis also pointed to the contradiction experienced by those workers who are promoted to management, including nurse managers. Giddens (1989) states that, according to Eric Olin Wright, such promotions position these workers in a contradiction or contradictory class location. Within Marxist understandings they belong to the working class, but are presumed to now carry out the wishes of the dominating class. The term "contradiction" does not admit that this managerial class might also act in the interests of workers, or more importantly, attempt to act in the interests of both classes. It is this idea that we wish to explore in relation to nurse managers, extending the idea that nurse managers act in the interests of the state, the patients, and staff nurses. Our argument is that nurse managers are in a position to use technology in the interest of the state, technology in the care of patients, and technology in the contradictory interests or care of staff nurses.

CONTEMPORARY CRITICISMS OF NURSING LABOR AND TECHNOLOGY

Critiques of Fordist and neo-Fordist developments in nursing over the last decade have taken two distinct but related paths. Both have been highly critical of nurse managers or hospital administrators. First, Brannon (1990, 1994), commenting on the North American experience, has been critical of primary nursing and its promise of neo-Fordist work arrangements, specifically, the reunification of nursing tasks. Brannon (1990, 1994) argues that while the shift to primary nursing overcomes the division of labor where untrained staff and lower-level or auxiliary nurses do most of the hands-on care, including the emotional labor, and while registered nurses do the more technical and managerial labor, the gains have been two-edged. Registered nurses now often find themselves responsible for total patient care in units that are understaffed (read cost-saving or profit-making), and where there is no one to whom tasks may be delegated.

In the examples cited by Brannon (1990), it was clear that managers had not changed the staff mix only in the interests of task unification, but rather, because it was cheaper to employ nurses who were registered to perform all the technical tasks than it was to employ a mix of various grades of nurses, many of whom were not qualified to handle the technology. While we would agree with Brannon's analysis, we would argue that it is simplistic to suggest that management has only one interest: cost containment. Decisions about the organization of nursing work are made in an environment where there are a number of interests, with nurse managers engaging in a process of weighing up benefits and costs to staff. Brannon (1990) stated that staff nurses could see the benefits of reorganization; however, his later (1994) review notes the shift back to team nursing as managers come to see its economic benefits.

The second critique, taken up by commentators such as Campbell (1992), writing on health care reform in Canada, is critical of the way nursing has embraced electronic and digital technologies and collaborated with management. She suggests that nurses have been too quick to assist management in innovating and finding ways to deal with budgetary cuts and restructuring. This has often been done through using computer technology on the wards to record bed occupancy or nursing hours. In cooperating with management, this knowledge moves from nursing knowledge to management control. It is also of a technical kind, so that nursing tasks may be timed and measured, but the subtle work of nursing, including emotional labor, remains unrecorded on computer-generated staffing programs. Campbell's analysis suggests that technology increases Taylorist forms of control, since it reduces nursing labor to a set of tasks where management controls the mental side, while staff nurses do the physical or manual side.

BELAIR SERVICES: A CASE STUDY IN THE RESTRUCTURING PROCESS

In the opening paragraphs we outlined the care offered by Belair Services and detailed one small innovation introduced into the organization. In 1994, Belair Services underwent an external review motivated by budget shortfalls, the de-institutionalization movement, and developments within both the private and government sectors for best practice (Morris, 1996). This review identified low levels of client satisfaction and suggested that legislated standards of care were not being consistently met. An internal review of nursing services in 1995 identified disproportionately high levels of staff in comparison to other organizations similarly placed, and resulted in the State Health Commission calling for a reduction in nursing hours from an average of 8 to 2.8 and 6.0 hours per client day in the two major areas. The issue for nurse managers was to examine the appropriateness of the recommended reduction in hours for quality nursing care. In addition, they had to "fight" to keep the institution open in the interests of a number of clients who did not want to be "integrated into the community," and in the interests of the numerous staff nurses committed to the care of these residents who wished to retain their jobs.

As a result of intensive examination of all nursing practices, a wide range of strategies was implemented under the direction of nursing management. In four years the nursing staffing levels were decreased from around 500 full-time equivalent (FTE) to 300 FTE and nursing hours per client to 6 and 4 hours per day. This was achieved through offering redeployment for nursing staff to other institutions and through voluntary redundancy packages. No staff were forcibly retrenched. Ancillary workers were employed to do "non-nursing" duties formerly carried out by nurses, such as collecting medications from the pharmacy and transporting clients to clinic appointments. Part of the restructuring process involved the introduction of new technologies through a process of evidenced-based nursing care. One example of the new technologies introduced is the electronic beds and lifting equipment mentioned above. Two examples are detailed below: an automated rostering system and the purchase of continence devices.

It became apparent that the "peaks and troughs" of nursing activity were not satisfactorily addressed. For example, the lowest activity time on many wards was 2:30 P.M.–3:30 P.M., when the maximum number of nurses were on duty due to an overlap in the two-day shifts. A complex variety of shift configurations was required. This was achieved through the acquisition, installation, and implementation of an automated rostering system, which enabled nurse unit managers to allocate the maximum number of staff to peak activity times such as early morning and meal times. This resulted in significant savings in staffing overall, and also increased the number of staff available at peak activity times. Client incidents, once significantly higher at meal times, decreased, as well as overall client satisfaction with the nursing service. Here is an example of technology used in the interest of flexibility, but this flexibility may not have been in the interest of nursing staff who had to accommodate to new shift arrangements.

Nursing innovations were not confined to rostering systems that "controlled" the labor process of nurses. As would be expected with the client group, the management of continence is a significant issue for the organization. Contemporary nursing practices were not being well utilized prior to the review, with significant numbers of clients requiring full linen changes every two to four hours. The employment of a full-time Continence Nurse Adviser led to the individualized assessment of all clients with continence issues, and radical changes to continence management, including the purchase of appropriate continence devices for clients according to need. Contemporary practices continue, and although the cost of continence products has increased significantly, the cost of linen has decreased, resulting in a net saving. The corresponding decrease in the amount of time nurses now spend changing wet beds, and the enhanced dignity and comfort of clients, demonstrated the efficacy of using the new products.

CONTRADICTIONS IN THE RESTRUCTURING PROCESS

Each of the innovations and accompanying technologies was introduced into Belair Services as a result of the endeavors of nurse managers working with nurses on the wards. Technology has enhanced nursing practices within the organization and created the capacity for nurses to focus their efforts on higher-level caring activities such as assessment, monitoring client outcomes, and communication. However, as suggested in the introduction, this was done within the context of restructuring where some technologies increased management control over nursing labor, shifted work from one grade of worker to another, or resulted in redeployment. Are we now to address emancipation only for clients, and not for nurses? Or is care always service toward the "other" at the expense of the "self?"

A simplistic answer would be to suggest that the technologies be separated out, with those benefiting clients embraced and those with ambiguous advantages to nurses more carefully examined. However, health-related technologies are not so easily categorized, as the case of the hydraulic beds demonstrates. The relationship between any technology, work, and capitalist social relations appears to always serve the interests of owners or the state, even if it also serves the interests of patients and possibly the interests of workers. Further, labor-saving devices are rarely wholly liberating, since as we suggested above, technology is not used simply to free humans from labor, but is also used to increase profits (efficiencies) for owners, managers, and shareholders. Also, human labor can be intensified concurrently with the introduction of time-saving technology, as many workers in Western countries are now discovering.

However, it is also simplistic to suggest that nurse managers act only in the interests of owners or the state, particularly in state-funded health care facilities where industrial protection for all levels of workers is still reasonably robust and where the managers themselves still identify as caring nurses. Each of the technological changes introduced into Belair

Services was done in the interests of both clients and staff nurses: Management that saw itself as engaging in the task of juggling a shrinking budget; a health department that wished to solve the problem by closing the institution down; a client base that deserved quality care; and a group of caring nurses who wished to retain their jobs. It is possible to bring a critical analysis to these processes, but it is simplistic to assume that managers are not aware of the contradictions, both of the efficiencies and of care for clients. The dilemma for nurse managers is how to manage the contradictions.

REFERENCES

Abercrombie, N., Hill, S., & Turner, B. (1984). *Dictionary of Sociology*. London: A. Lane.

Brannon, R. (1990). The professionalization of the nursing labor process: From team to primary nursing. *International Journal of Health Services, 20*, 511–524.

Brannon, R. (1994). Professionalization and work intensification. *Work and Occupations, 21*, 157–178.

Braverman, H. (1974). *Labor and monopoly capitalism*. New York: Monthly Review Press.

Campbell, M. (1992). Nurses' professionalism in Canada: A labor process analysis. *International Journal of Health Services, 22*, 751–765.

Cheek, J., Shoebridge, J., Willis, E., & Zadoroznyj, M. (1996). *Society and health: Social theory for health workers*. Sydney: Longman.

Giddens, A. (1989). *Sociology*. London: Polity Press.

Hsiao, W. (1992). What nations can learn from one another. *Journal of Health Politics, Policy and Law, 17*, 613–636.

Mathews, J. (1992). New Production systems—A response to critics and a re-evaluation. *Australian Journal of Political Economy, 30*, 91–128.

Morris, R. (1996). The age of workplace reform in Australia. In D. Mortimer, P. Leece, & R. Morris (Eds.), *Workplace reform and enterprise bargaining* (pp. 11–24). Sydney: Harcourt Brace.

Waters, M., & Crook, S. (1993). *Sociology one: Principles of sociological analysis*. Melbourne: Longman Cheshire.

Chapter 15

Demand Pull or Technology Push: Which Is Influencing Change in Nursing Care and Information Practice?

P. Jane Greaves and Stephen Wilmot

INTRODUCTION

The ongoing debate among health care professionals about the determinants of technology and technological change, and their relationship to the delivery of high-quality care, proceeds apace. Some would like to think that nursing care is changing, and the quality of nursing care and information improving due to the technological demands and decisions nurses are making.

This chapter explores theories of technological determinism and the demand pull, technology push issue which Freeman (1987) identified as an ill-structured debate among economists and historians of science and technology. Demand pull and technology push issues are influencing the way nursing care can be delivered and managed by nurses. Technology, not nursing, may be the active force which is changing current care practices and influencing the professional values of care which have underpinned nursing for so long.

This chapter explores both the hardware-led theory of technological determinism and the theory of soft technological determinism, and how these concepts, not nursing, may be the active force which is causing change today. Nursing has a responsibility on a national and international basis to make sure its voice is clearly heard among the incessant chatter of information technology (IT) spin doctors, as the effective design and implementation of computerized information systems which nurses can use is predicated on nursing's information and caring needs, and not necessarily on those of business alone.

It is also incumbent on organizations that govern and represent nursing to be proactive in making sure nursing's needs are clearly met in advance of system design and implementation, so that quality care, determined by the values that underpin nursing practice, can be delivered. Expecting each individual practitioner to engage in rational choice decision making with regard to caring and information technology, when they are only in possession of the barest facts and knowledge of such systems, is naive in the extreme, in the face of such powerful forces for change as the current IT revolution in health care. Freeman's suggestion (1987) is still valid today, that the push from technologists who wish to promote technical advance is hard for society to resist, as new applications for these developments are identified continuously. Nursing's slow recognition of the new paradigm of information-intensive, flexible, computerized technology, and lack of involvement in the technological push which is changing health care today seriously threatens the caring philosophy that underpins nursing care delivery. Turkle (1987) suggests that the use of computers provides nurses with unprecedented opportunities and with unprecedented risks as technology catalyses change, not only in what we do but in how we think. The potential of such pervasive technology to influence change in all areas of health care practice cannot be ignored, and clearly requires more of our attention. The nursing profession has a responsibility to make sure its voice is clearly heard in the arena of health informatics, and to be proactive in the development of IT systems that meet their professional requirements. As Senn (1990) suggests, if we do not play a role in the development of IT systems, we will have no choice but to accept the decisions others make for us.

TECHNOLOGICAL DETERMINISM

Technological determinism assumes that social development is achieved by technology alone and that technology is the active force causing change. Although there is no precise meaning for the term "technological determinism," it would be useful to explore the concept in relation to the introduction and use of technology and computerized systems by nurses.

There are two main theories of technological determinism: First, the Hardware-led Theory, which suggests that social change is determined by an autonomous technology which is self-standing and independent of social shaping. The initial development of computers and information technology for business and military purposes could have been said to have been revolutionary in its introduction, development, and continuing impact on all aspects of work and communications. The eventual use of this medium within the health care environment would appear, in hindsight, to have been inevitable, and now pervades all areas of practice, including nursing. Computers and information technology within nursing constitute a radical innovation and have required new rules, practices, and customs to be developed which differ considerably from the previously prevailing paradigm suggested by Stonham (1999) as actions which were largely professionally contained and autonomous, resulting in care and treatment which suffered from lack of integration, untimely and disjointed delivery, and fragmented communication. But the quantum leap in potential productivity made possible by the introduction and use of new technologies, Freeman (1987) suggests, cannot easily be realized without considerable organizational and social change of far-reaching character. Miller and MacIntosh (1994) observed that the introduction and implementation of information systems were taking place at a time of rapid, continuous, and complex change in health care. This exercise was being colored by historical management styles, resistance to change, imposition of external requirements rather than local choice in the decision-making process, and the lack of appropriate specifications of what a nursing information system should comprise. One has to wonder, with this sort of scenario, how much nurses are getting involved in the development of these systems; but regardless of resistance, nursing and health care practice are changing. The development of modern IT systems within nursing is happening unchecked at a lightning pace, and nursing practice is being required to accommodate its needs accordingly. This would appear to support the Hardware-led Theory. If this belief is held, it makes the development of IT systems in nursing and health care easy to explain, encouraging the idea that predictions about future planning, development, use, and control by nurses can and will be made. Newell (1998) suggested that doctors required considerable change in working practice and procedures both to enable efficient implementation of clinical systems and also to realize organizational benefits. There is no reason to suppose that nursing will be any different.

Social intervention in the hardware-led process has been shown to soften its impact, through the influence of policy makers' values and aims in systems design, suggests Kling (1987), and this acknowledges that social and human factors can influence the use and effectiveness of technology in the caring environment. The theory of Soft Technological Determinism also views technology as the primary cause of change, but takes account of social factors in the way of anticipating barriers, both physical and psychological, that may obstruct the introduction and efficient use of such technologies as computerized health care information systems. However, acknowledgment of the social factors that may influence technologies is tempered by the fact that it is a recognition that there may be a reaction to, rather than an impact on, the implementation and development of these technologies. It does not acknowledge that there will or should be proactive involvement of nurses in the decision-making process that shapes the development of such technologies. The assumption is that technology is the active force causing change, and social and human factors play only a passive role, following behind whereever each innovation leads, resistance being overcome by user education, preparation, and forward planning.

Evidence of the technology push can clearly be identified in nursing as we continue to spend valuable time entering data into systems which provide limited relevant information for nurses actually engaged in delivering care. It is no surprise, then, that Reeve and Wheeler (1995) stated, "nurses do not hold computerized information to be of any intrinsic value either to themselves or their patients" (p. 30). This view is supported by Cooper (1999), who suggests that many nurses do not consider IT of any use to them, and are concerned about having systems imposed upon them that they believe do not contain any real benefits for them or their patients.

The technology push/pull scenario was implied by Robertson (1998) when discussing the process of modeling care in order to prevent the influence of technology, requiring us to alter care practices for no obvious benefit. Nurses must get involved in defining their information needs, and ensuring that any solutions people try to sell them really do meet their professional needs, in other words, a "demand-pull" by nurses to guarantee their needs are met.

However, the explanatory benefits of technological determinism on this issue may be outweighed by the limitations of its deterministic nature. Technological determinism is a version of the philosophical position of determinism. Determinists take the view that individual agency and responsibility are illusions, because the reality is that all events and all human actions are determined. All are part of a causal chain which can in theory be predicted, and is therefore determined. This leaves no room for the unpredictability of individual choice. Nineteenth-century physical sciences framed material processes as propelled by the unilinear and unidirectional cause–effect sequences typical of nineteenth-century mechanics, and therefore often termed "mechanistic." This provided the basis for the determinist view, and contributed to pessimism about human agency in such divergent perspectives as Marxism and psychoanalysis.

Technological determinism replaces the traditional determinist's mechanistic view of physics with a mechanistic view of technological development, determined by laws which cannot be changed by human decision; and because it applies the same principles, albeit to a different area, it is vulnerable to the same counterarguments as traditional determinism. Capra (1984) argues that technological determinism encourages a view that "technology determines the nature of our value system and our social relations, rather than recognizing that it is the other way round; that our values and social relations determine the nature of our technology" (p. 230). Warnock (1998) argues that the human mind (and therefore human behavior) cannot be drawn into a determinist causal chain because the multiple levels of explanation necessary to explain mental processes are, by their nature, complex beyond conceivable prediction. However, at a more fundamental level, mechanistic determinism is based on an erroneous view of science. The causal predictions of science are based on probability, not certainty, and the human sciences are particularly dependent on a sometimes tenuous degree of probability. In fact, the most fundamental of the physical sciences, physics, is characterized at certain levels by considerable uncertainty, so the nineteenth-century model of mechanistic science is, in any case, obsolete. So whether we see the development of technology as molded by human behavior or by the behavior of the technology itself, there is no secure philosophical basis for technological determinism. However, this does not necessarily solve the problems that deterministic thinking is likely to create in this area. A belief that certain processes are inevitable will become self-fulfilling, as those who could act otherwise decide that they have no choice. Determinism as an ideology can be profoundly disempowering, even though it is philosophically unsound.

OTHER EXPLANATIONS

Determinism seeks to predict, whereas what is required is explanation. It is necessary, indeed empowering, to explain why technology should be such a powerful force in the development of IT in health care. On the other side of the equation, the response of nurses to technology needs explaining. An explanation for the apathy that nurses show toward involvement in shaping IT systems may be found in some theories of social change when applied to nursing. A form of structuralism emphasizes that individual choices and decisions are influenced by a combination of interrelated, institutional forces. For example, the effects of gender socialization, nurse education, the health care industry and market forces, and individual professional symbols and values, none of which are autonomous in their own right, all have an impact on a predominantly female profession. Supporters of a structuralist theory consider that successful utilization and development of multiple forms of technology only take place after a period of change and adaptation of many social institutions to the new requirements of technology has occurred. There is usually a great deal of inertia in social institutions, buttressed by political power of established interest groups as well as slow response times of many individuals and groups (Freeman, 1987).

This seems a convincing argument when applied to health care professionals in Britain, and British nurses in particular. Practitioners in some areas of care appear comfortable with the use of highly sophisticated forms of technology to deliver and manage care, yet others continue to deliver care in much the same way as they have for many years. In both respects, nursing has only responded to the technology either in accepting it or rejecting it; it has not engaged in shaping and developing it for the benefit of patients and the delivery of improvements in care quality.

Such structural explanations, while not deterministic, may in a more limited way be disempowering for nurses in dealing with IT. The identification of general structural constraints, relating to gender, professional culture, market forces, and so on, creates a sense of the individual being a helpless pawn in the face of powerful forces; and yet, such explanations cast light on the process and need to be considered. So here we have a dilemma. Structural explanations cannot be refuted as can determinism, and they have something to tell nurses; but it is difficult for individual nurses to find an empowered response to the processes they identify.

An acknowledgment of interactive processes in society—particularly of conflict and competition—offers the individual actor a more significant role. Such a perspective would emphasize the conflicts of competition, control, and power inherent in human society. We can see that the development of information technology in health care has been radically influenced by certain groups to exert professional or managerial control over other groups. For example, Greaves (1998) suggests that many nurses working alongside general practitioners (GPs) in Britain are deprived of appropriate or any IT training. This may be because GPs rather than nurses control the training budget. Consequently, although the potential is there for nurses to improve the quality of service they can provide, their ability to fulfill this need is compromised through lack of training. As Murry (1994) states, "computer use in nursing is littered with false starts and broken promises" (p. 27).

The choice of technology and the way it is applied to care delivery are a political issue, because the purposes of employers are not necessarily consonant with those of nurses or other health care professionals. The use of these systems is often said to provide greater professional autonomy and empowerment for nurses, but many have found in industry that the rhetoric of empowerment is used only to intensify work through the measurement of mean times for interaction and imposing these as standards. This has been evident in some commercial operator call centers in Britain and the United States, and nurses should be aware of these pressures as the "NHS direct" health care call centers continue to develop (Department of Health, 1997). Areas of IT that cannot be used for these ends are less likely to be financed or developed.

THE WAY FORWARD FOR NURSING

It is clear that the nurse's position is not much more comfortable in the competitive situation described in the previous paragraph than it is in the mechanistic universe of the determinist. However, nurses have the option of engaging in that competitive arena, and they have a value-base that potentially enables them to do this, despite structural constraints of gender and professional culture. Wilmot (1993) argues that the value placed on individual autonomy, agency, and responsibility in nursing provides a counterweight to the disempowering impact of deterministic thinking in the physical and social sciences. However, that counterweight has arguably not been fully realized in nurse education or nursing practice. There is a need for a two-pronged response to the problem of technological determinism. On the one hand, the ideology of deterministic passivity, which taps into a psychology of helplessness, needs to be combated in the culture of nursing; and the ideology of individual agency and responsibility in nursing needs to be renewed and refreshed for the new situation. Wurzbach (1999) argues that autonomy is one of the most powerful moral metaphors in the discourse of nursing, but it can only be sustained in professional discourse if it is sustainable in practice. A repertoire of practical IT skills is necessary to do this. Only by having a command of the technology can the individual nurse come to see that Capra was right; that our values and social relations really do determine the nature of our technology, and that the technology can be the servant of the values.

In conclusion, it can be seen that technological determinism has had a malign influence on explanations of the development of IT. The argument that technology is synonymous with progress and progress is inevitable is profoundly disempowering to all human service professionals. In the new millennium, nursing historians may look back on the growth of computing as one of the most important factors that influenced changes in care management and delivery, and the professional development and actions of nurses. If this is so, one has to ask why, as one of the largest groups of people working toward a caring society, and actively involved in the delivery of quality care, are we not more intimately involved in the design and development of IT systems?

Nurses and their professional values and needs, rather than technology alone, should determine the development of new forms of technology and IT which facilitate the delivery of high-quality care. Consequently, technological determinism should be resisted by the nursing profession, as it has the power to change the very nature of nursing care practice and encourages a narrow view of a very complex activity.

REFERENCES

Capra, F. (1984). *The turning point: Science, society and the rising culture*. London: Fontana.

Cooper, C. (1999). Jottings from the chair. *Information Technology in Nursing, 11*(2), 4–5.

Department of Health. (1997). *The new NHS: Modern, dependable*. London: HMSO.

Freeman, C. (1987). The case for technological determinism. In R. Finnegan, G. Salaman, & K. Thompson (Eds.), *Information technology: Social issues*. London: Hodder and Stoughton.

Greaves, P. J. (1998). Nurses' knowledge of patient information security in health care information systems: A cause for concern. In B. Richards (Ed.), *Current perspectives in health care computing: Conference proceedings* (pp. 77–84). Surrey, England: Harrogate, BJHC & BCS.

Kling, R. (1987). Value conflicts and social choice in electronic payment systems. In R. Finnegan, G. Salaman, & K. Thompson (Eds.), *Information technology: Social issues*. London: Hodder and Stoughton.

Miller, A., and MacIntosh, J. (1994). Use and abuse of NIS. In G. Wright & D. Evans (Eds.), *Sharing information: Focusing on the patient*. Conference proceedings. Leicestershire: British Computer Society Nursing Specialist Group.

Murry, P. J. (1994). Hyper CAL: Hypertext is the future for nurse education to develop their own courseware. In *IT—Supporting Professional Education Conference*. English National Board, National Board of Scotland, Edinburgh.

Newell, J. (1998). Clinical computing: Tacking stock, looking forward. *The British Journal of Health Care Computing and Information Management, 15*(5), 24–26.

Reeve, J., and Wheeler, S. (1995). The silent barrier. *The British Journal of Healthcare Computing and Information Management, 12*(8), 35–37.

Robertson, I. (1998). Modeling the process of health visiting. *Information Technology in Nursing, 10*(1), 19.

Senn, J. (1990). *Information systems in management* (4th ed.). Belmont, CA: Wadsworth.

Stonham, G. (1999). Changing healthcare delivery with IT. *Information Technology in Nursing, 9*(6), 16–17.

Turkle, S. (1987). Computers and the human spirit. In R. Finnegan, G. Salaman, & K. Thompson (Eds.), *Information technology: Social issues*. London: Hodder and Stoughton.

Warnock, M. (1998). *An intelligent person's guide to ethics*. London: Duckworth.

Wilmot, S. (1993). Ethics, agency and empowerment in nurse education. *Nurse Education Today, 13*(3), 189–195.

Wurzbach, M. (1999). The moral metaphors of nursing. *Journal of Advanced Nursing, 30* (1), 94–99.

Chapter 16

Exploring the Gender-Technology Relation in Nursing

Margarete Sandelowski

INTRODUCTION

Feminist and nursing scholars have emphasized the crucial role Western technology has played in the history and development of women and nursing; feminists most concerned with the gender-technology relation and nurses most concerned with the nursing-technology relation. Yet, despite their common ground in tying both the emancipation and the subordination of women and nurses to technology, there had been virtually no association between nursing and gender-technology studies. This may be due, in part, to the mutual disdain nurses and feminists have felt for each other, the suspicion some nurses feel toward theories outside of nursing to resolve problems in nursing, and the cultural devaluation of the feminine that affects them both. Nursing is too female for many feminists, while feminism is not female enough for some nurses (Baer, 1991; Fagin, 1994; Gordon, 1991; Roberts & Group, 1995).

In this chapter I offer the outlines of a theoretical and research association between nursing and gender-technology studies, and suggest how it might be mutually beneficial to the advancement of both these fields. In short, I propose that the field of gender-technology studies offers nursing scholars new analytic directions and methodological tools to explore the nursing-technology relation. Nursing, in turn, offers the field of gender-technology studies a rich empirical site to further its theoretical development.

GENDER-TECHNOLOGY STUDIES: ANALYTIC
DIRECTIONS AND TOOLS FOR NURSING

Gender-technology studies are an interdisciplinary field of scholarship that emerged in the late 1970s, from the social science critique of Western science and technology, and the feminist critique of the academic disciplines and professions that began in the 1960s (Traweek, 1993). Drawing primarily from history, sociology, and cultural studies, scholars in the field have taken on several projects ranging from the liberal feminist goal of ensuring women's equal access to technology fields, to the more radical feminist agenda of exposing the negative effects of technological innovations on women. More recently, gender-technology scholars have sought to theorize the Western cultural association between technology and masculinity. The increasing use of the term "gender studies" (as opposed to feminist critique) of technology signals a more serious effort to study gender as a cultural construction implicating both women and men (as opposed to studying only women). Contemporary studies that make problematic the gender-technology relation, however, remain informed by largely feminist, or pro-women, liberatory goals (Grint & Gill, 1995; Kirkup & Keller, 1992; Wajcman, 1991; Woolgar, 1995).

Gender-technology scholars have emphasized the underrepresentation of women in technology fields, and also their misrepresentation as only users, but not inventors, of technology. They have shown that women were more than footnotes in the history of technology, by documenting their contributions to agriculture and food production, health and medicine, sex and reproduction, and machine and computer technologies. They have also examined the structural, psychological, and sociocultural factors that have impeded women's inventive capacity, motivation, and opportunity, including educational, occupational, and economic barriers to women in technology fields; and their access to public and commercial rewards for invention. Gender-technology scholars have also exposed the often negative effects not only of technologies used largely or exclusively by women (such as household and reproductive technologies), but also of ostensibly gender-neutral technologies, such as computers. Current efforts in the field are directed toward explaining the nature, ethics, and politics of the Western cultural association between technology and masculinity. Scholars increasingly seek to understand how gender and technology are constitutive of each other; how Western technology embodies or consolidates masculine identity, practices, and values; and how technology can be an equalizer in societies characterized by gender, class, and race inequalities (Cowan, 1983; Faulkner & Arnold, 1985; Harney, 1993; Hynes, 1991; McGaw, 1982; Perry, 1990; Ratcliff, 1989; Rothschild,

1983, 1988; Spallone & Steinberg, 1987; Stanley, 1995; Stanworth, 1987; Trescott, 1979).

THE NURSING-TECHNOLOGY RELATION

Since the beginnings of modern nursing in the latter half of the nineteenth century, nurses have addressed the material world of practice and the practical problems of "nursing the equipment" (Smith, 1932) and the patient. Before the widespread use of machine technology in the late 1950s, nurses were primarily concerned with maintaining and making the best of the devices available to them to comfort and treat patients (Sandelowski, 1997a). After 1960, nurses were concerned with learning the intricacies of the "new machinery" (Harris, 1966) for monitoring and with its potential to replace nursing. By the 1980s, nurses were asking whether and how new technologies, which redefined and extended living, dying, and the traditional watchful vigilance of the nurse, were ethically compatible with nursing touch and humanistic nursing care. Now, at the beginning of the twenty-first century, nurses continue to address the (ir)reconcilability of technology with nursing care, and to contrast *high-tech* and *high-touch* care (Sandelowski, 1997b).

As this very abbreviated history of the nursing-technology relation indicates, nurses have always been in some ways concerned with how technology influences both the practice and (re)presentation of nursing as an academic and caring profession. Such devices as the stethoscope, sphygmomanometer, and pulse oximeter have been used as "aesthetically less complicated and culturally-resonant means to signify or portray nursing" (Walker, 1994, p. 52). Whether it was the craft technology that largely characterized nursing practice before World War II, or the computer technologies that characterize it now, technology has been central to debates concerning the relationship between hands, mind, and spirit of the nurse; and the representation of nursing as a fine performance art; basic, applied, or practical science; or as a (woman) craft.

What the gender-technology studies offer nursing are new definitions of and orientations to technology, and new and, arguably, the right questions to ask about the nursing-technology relation. Lawler (1991) observed that the questions asked about and in nursing have often served only to further silence nurses and/or marginalize nursing. Gender-technology studies may offer nurses away to be heard and nursing a way to be seen at the center of health care.

Redefining Technology

Gender-technology scholars have sought to create more inclusive definitions of technology. Feminist critics have noted that prevailing definitions of technology have emphasized technologies of primary interest to men, rather than those associated with female lives and work. *Masculine* inventions, such as cars, bombs, and computers, are seen as not only technology but also as both spectacular and significant. *Feminine* technologies, such as menstrual hygiene products, baby bottles, and washing machines, disappear from view as *Technology* and, along with them, the opportunity to study critical roles they have played in women's history and development (Stanley, 1995; Trescott, 1979; Wajcman, 1991).

Nurses have tended also not to see the everyday and familiar things in their practice words as constituting technology (Fairman, 1992), reserving that term for more spectacular devices such as electronic monitors and ultrasound machines. Yet, the devices used to bathe, purge, and catheterize patients not only constitute technology, but are significant technology in the history of nursing and health care. A special case in point is the bed. Nursing has historically been theorized and imaged as occurring at the bedside. For most of nursing history, the greatest part of the nurse's work was "around, about, and with the bed" (Harmer, 1922, p. 33). Moreover, patients were often confined for weeks and months in bed.

Nurses' and patients' relation to beds changed dramatically as new medical technologies (including pharmaceuticals and surgery) permitted patients to get out of bed sooner, and as new electrical and electronic beds permitted patients more control over their movements in bed. Nurses' physical labor associated with the bedridden patient was also reduced with new bed designs and associated technologies, such as hydraulic lifts. Yet, a new kind of labor associated with the newly mobile and ambulatory patient replaced the hard work of manually cranking beds and lifting patients into proper position. Ambulatory patients posed surveillance and safety issues that bedridden patients had not. Moreover, while patients were getting up out of bed, nurses themselves were literally and figuratively moving away from it. Nurses increasingly delegated bedside nursing activities to other, ancillary personnel.

In short, the bed has been a focal point around which much that is crucial in nursing history has occurred. Arguably, the bed, as fact and symbol of nursing and the care of the sick, has been a contested terrain, as physicians, nurses, and their delegates have sought to gain access to it, control activities around it, but not to spend too much time, or be defined, by it. Nursing history can be read, in part, as a consent for and/ or abandonment of the bed (Lynaugh, 1989, 1994). Yet, the bed has received virtually no attention at all as a significant technology. Little attention has been paid to how design changes in hospital and patient beds have reflected, influenced, or even configured nursing practices. Among the many questions that have yet to be answered are: What assumptions about user and use are revealed in the actual physical form the hospital bed has taken over time? Was it assumed that women would be the primary users of these beds, or were they designed from the vantage point of patients? Was there any connection between changes in bed designs and the increased mobility of patients? Did bed technology influence nurses' views of patients? What social relations and divisions of labor did bed technology engender among patients, nurses, physicians, and others? The bed is a familiar and ostensibly gender-neutral technology, which, on closer inspection through the lens of gender-technology studies, appears not so neutral at all. Victorian debates about women's proper role in and out of the home were manifested in and influenced by different sewing machine designs (Douglas, 1982). Nineteenth- and twentieth-century debates about what constituted proper care of the premature infant and appropriate roles for mothers, nurses, and physicians in that care were manifested in and shaped by infant incubator designs (Baker, 1996). Changes in the hospital bed may offer similar information about nursing.

Rethinking the Technology-Science Relation

Gender-technology scholars have emphasized the controversial relations between technology and science. Nurses have tended to view technology as "simply the application of science" (Jacox, 1992, p. 70). Yet, the findings from gender (and other social science and cultural) studies of technology indicate that there is nothing simple about the relationship between science and technology, and that it is simplistic to conceive of technology solely as the material outcome of science. In current models of the science-technology relation, science and technology are distinguishable subcultures and knowledge fields, with technological innovation seen as the key factor in the seventeenth-century Western revolution. Instead of technology solely being dependent on science, modern Western science is a largely visual enterprise, dependent on technologies (such as the telescope, microscope, and ultrasound machine) that allow scientists to see the nature they subsequently reconstruct as science. Moreover, all technology has historically maintained a close relationship to art and craft by virtue of its emphasis on design, non-verbal practices, aesthetic vision, and skilled making (Sandelowski, 1997c).

The new primacy of technology over science and technology gives new visibility and priority to nursing practices that involve complex interplays between knowing *that* and knowing *how*. Because many nursing practices cannot readily be languaged, they have remained invisible and therefore unrecognized as constituting knowledge (Parker & Gardner, 1992; Wolf, 1989). Nursing manual, visual, and other non-verbal knowledges have often been dismissed as not-knowledge; that is, as simply the robotic completion of procedures following physicians' orders. Viewed from the vantage point of the nursing-technology relation, the knowledge needed to order the application of an electronic fetal monitor, for example, is no more valuable or complex than the knowledge needed to produce an accurate recording of fetal heart rate and uterine contraction patterns and to maintain women's safety and comfort. These activities require practice theories of intervention, approach, deliberation, and enactment (Kim, 1994); they require particularized and "practically practical" knowledge to direct concrete action, as opposed to general and "speculative" knowledge of things to be done (Bottorff, 1991; Johnson, 1991). In their long-standing efforts to make nursing over into a *thinking* academic discipline, nurses have arguably been reluctant to explore and theorize the *practical* in nursing, for fear of reinstating a view of nursing as solely defined by procedures.

The new, analytic emphasis on technology as a distinctive domain of knowledge that includes embodied ways of knowing may also lead nursing scholars to confront and even arrest the nursing flight from the body, the traditional site of these procedures and, historically, "pivotal concern for the practice of nursing" (Lawler, 1991, p. 4). Indeed, one important kind of human-technology relation in nursing is an epistemic relation of embodiment, in which instrumentation extends to the senses and physical capacities of the nurse (Ihde, 1979; Sandelowski, 1997c). The denial of the body work of nursing is evident both in theoretical efforts to place nursing on an intellectual plane equal to other academic and scientific disciplines, and in the practice of increasingly delegating body work to ancillary personnel. The problem of the body in nursing, as Lawler (1991) insightfully described it, is partly a result of the configuration of knowledge that excludes the body (p. 3). A key characteristic of this configuration in Western thought is the subordination of the artistic and manual to the intellectual and verbal, and resulting subordination of technology to science (Ferguson, 1977). Although the actual practice of nursing necessarily and inevitably concerns the body (Lawler, 1991), scientific abstractions of nursing knowledge minimize it. Both Lawler (1991) and Wolf (1986) argued that body work is tainted in Western culture as women's work and dirty work. Technology is a distinctive way of knowing persons that provides space to theorize further the links between gender and body work (Lawler, 1991). This body work has traditionally included technologies for bathing, feeding, and comforting that have, like the bed, yet to draw much attention as significant technologies.

Avoiding Determinism and Essentialism

In addition to offering more expansive views of technology and the technology-science relation, gender-technology scholars have sought to move beyond deterministic and essentialistic explanations of gender and technology (Berg & Lie, 1995; Grint & Woolgar, 1995). Technological determinism is a view of technology as a neutral and first cause of, and therefore separate form of, social change. Technology is conceived as an *It* uninformed by, but having effects and impact on, society and culture, largely owing to its technical features. Technological progress is viewed linearly and is inevitably leading to certain inventions and designs. Essentialism is a kind of deterministic explanation in which unvarying characteristics are attributed to persons or entities. That is, Feminine, Masculine, and Technology are each depicted as having essences essentially untouched by history or culture. For example, in some eco-feminist critiques of technology, an eternal and constant feminine nature is viewed as being in opposition to masculine technology (Gill & Grint, 1995).

Like many feminist critics of technology, nurses have tended toward deterministic and essentialistic arguments to explore the nursing-technology relation. They have tended not to differentiate among the many and diverse health/medical technologies and, instead, have merged these technologies into monolithic *Technology*, which, in turn, is conceived as an *It* having positive and/or negative effects on nursing (Sandelowski, 1997c). The essentializing of technology may also reflect a problem of language, as opposed to conceptualization. As Grint and Woolgar (1995) observed, as "prisoners of the conventions of language and representation, we display, reaffirm, and sustain the basic premises of essentialism" (p. 299). English-language customs make it difficult to convey the human-technology relation as if it were an entity separate from humans exerting effects. Yet, while technology is necessarily about things, it is also about a dynamic process; namely, humans in interaction with things to achieve human desires and purposes, whereby both the things and the desires are constantly being reinvented (Sandelowski, 1997b).

Nurses adhere to an epistemology of identity (Annandale & Clark, 1996) when they take virtually no account of the differences (for example, in origin, purpose, design, operations, and use) among the vast array of technologies for diagnosis, therapy, and comfort. Moreover, there is a tendency in nursing to essentialize it as *Nursing*, which, in turn, is conceived as embodying feminine values in health care (such as caring and nurturance). In contrast, nurses adhere to an epistemology of difference when they place *Feminine Nursing* at odds with *Masculine Technology*.

Recent scholarship in gender-technology studies has been directed toward the anti-essentialistic aim of examining the commonalities and differences among the many femininities, masculinities, and technologies implicated in the gender-technology relation. Both gender and technology are increasingly conceived as constitutive of each other and reproduced in every social interaction. That is, there is no one Femininity, Masculinity, or Technology, but rather there are historically and culturally specific femininities, masculinities, and technologies. Depending on the context, gender is variously conceived as inextricable from, antecedent to, a condition for, and/or a consequence of, technological change. Technology is similarly variously conceived as inextricable from, antecedent to, a condition for, and/or a consequence of "doing gender" (West & Zimmerman, 1987). Gender is viewed here less as a dichotomous variable (Allen, Allman, & Powers, 1991) or an attribute of individuals who have gender, than, as West and Zimmerman put it, as an emergent feature of social situations (p. 126). Gender is both an outcome of and a rationale for various social arrangements. Gender is a continuing accomplishment, an achieved property of situated conduct, as opposed to a static property of individuals. Gender is not what a person is, but rather what she or he does. Like the making and doing of technology itself, doing gender is a kind of social performance. Doing gender means (re)creating differences between the sexes that are neither natural nor essential and, then, naturalizing and essentializing them.

Just as there are femininities, masculinities, and technologies, there are also historically and culturally specific *nursings*. Gender-technology studies direct nurses to consider the merits of an epistemology of identity, rather than of difference, leading them to ask: When is it useful to think of nursing as Nursing, or as comprised of historically and culturally situated, or specialty, nursings? When are distinctions made between nursing and technology, illuminating or deceptive, and emancipatory or regressive? (Gordon, 1991).

NURSING AS AN EMPIRICAL SITE FOR GENDER-TECHNOLOGY STUDIES

While gender-technology studies raise new questions for nurses to ask about nursing, nursing offers a rich empirical site for gender-technology studies (whether conducted by nurses or other scholars in that field).

A Site to Study Gender, Technology, and Equality

As one of the most sex-segregated and exploited domains of female work, nursing is an ideal venue to examine the democratizing potential of technology in conditions of gender inequality. By examining why technology has had so little effect in altering the social position of the nurse, gender-technology scholars will further their understanding of why the promise of new technological innovations to eliminate social inequalities so often fail women, and how these innovations might be harnessed for women's advancement. As a gender-marked (West & Zimmerman, 1987) group of professionals who share many of the same technologies with other gender-marked groups (medicine), nursing is an ideal site to study the different relations of women and men with the same technologies.

Technology has often been described as having emancipated women. For example, reproductive and housework technologies have been commonly viewed as leveling the educational and occupational playing field for women by eliminating or minimizing women's physical labor and many of the biological disadvantages associated with reproduction. Yet, gender-technology scholars have shown that reproductive and household technologies have also had the effect of reinforcing the gender norms that have traditionally assigned the greater burdens of housework and reproduction to women (Cowan, 1983; Ratcliff, 1989; Spallone & Steinberg, 1987; Stanworth, 1987). Most conceptive, contraceptive, and childbirth technologies are designed for use by women only, and they pose their own health risks of having sex and children. Women spend as much and even more time doing housework as they did before the advent of such devices as washing machines and vacuum cleaners. Moreover, the effect of some of these technological innovations has been to de-skill women in exercising their natural functions and to place them under the further control of men. A case in point is the early twentieth-century introduction of artificial infant feeding in the United States, which increasingly replaced breast-feeding and subjected mothers to the expertise and surveillance of physicians (Apple, 1987). Paradoxically, when looking at these *female* technologies, the more things have changed, the more they seem to have stayed the same.

Similarly, medical technology has been credited with both empowering and disempowering nurses. That is, scholars both in and out of nursing have viewed technology as expanding the sphere of influence of nursing. Nurses have gained valuable knowledge and skills that have made them indispensable to physicians and hospitals (Fairman, 1992; Melosh, 1982; Zalumas, 1995). Other scholars, however, have viewed medical technology as ultimately recirculating the traditionally unequal gender and professional relationships that have prevailed in health care (Hoffart, 1989; Koenig, 1988). Instead of expanding the sphere of influence of the nurse, technology has expanded the influence of the nurse over nursing, by maintaining control over access to technologies and by using nursing labor to achieve medical goals. Although both nurses and physicians have drawn much of their cultural authority and rewards from science and technology, nurses have not been similarly authorized or rewarded. Nurses still draw their authority largely from gender (including idealized notions of womanly caring and self-sacrifice), even while performing more and more of the work of technology in the hospital and, increasingly, in the home (Reverby, 1989). In the American health care system, physicians, but not nurses, are reimbursed for performing many of the same services (Griffith & Robinson, 1992).

A Site to Re(dis)cover Women's Contributions to Technology

Nursing is important also as an empirical site for the recovery of women's contributions to technological change. Nurses were essential to the technological transformation of hospitals of ostensibly *medical* technology. Nurses were key players in the late-nineteenth- and early-twentieth-century transformation of American hospitals into environments, not only conducive to healing (Rosenberg, 1987), but also into the "carefully established space [where were enacted] those rituals and ceremonies centered upon the conspicuous display of new tools and equipment" (Bledstein, 1976). Nurses made possible the advances in such highly technical domains as anesthesia, surgery, antisepsis, vital function monitoring, and intensive care. Indeed, the intensive care unit is better understood as an extension of the vigilance of private duty nursing than as a physical location for high concentrations of spectacular technologies (Fairman, 1992). The administration of anesthesia was originally a nursing, as opposed to a medical, specialty, as women were seen as especially suited to the work and to the lowly status (as compared to surgery, in physicians' eyes) of providing anesthesia (Bankert, 1989). Nurses were also increasingly relied on as the *soft* technology to counteract the depersonalizing impact of the new *hardware* entering hospitals. Primarily, nurses performed the "sentimental work in the technologized hospital" (Strauss et al., 1982, p. 254), by assisting reluctant and fearful patients to accept and accommodate to new technologies and by seeking to repair the damage to human dignity and autonomy that often accompanied technological change.

Nursing is also a key site for the rediscovery of female invention. Like other women, nurses remain hidden from history as inventors of health and medical technologies. From the earliest days of trained nursing, nurses have shown their inclinations and talents for altering the material of practice to enhance patient comfort, reduce nursing labor, and maximize nursing efficiency. Nurses worked to make the best of things available to them by transforming everyday and familiar objects into implements for comfort and healing. For example, in the earliest of trained nursing, they used bedside tables to relieve dyspnea, made bed supports for patients out of broom handles, and refashioned teapots and flower-sprinklers into enema cans (Sandelowski, 1997a). In the hands of these investigative nurses, everyday objects became "technological objects" (Ihde, 1990) in the domain of nursing.

Largely anecdotal evidence documents nurses' efforts to advise inventors and company detailmen on how to design new, and redesign exist-ing, devices. As the primary developers of technology in health care, nurses' advice has been crucial in the design of many devices and tech-nological systems; yet, few nurses are actually listed as patent holders themselves and few have received public recognition as inventors. More-over, because of their social position in health care and lack of training in, and alliances with, engineering and technology fields, nurses have not played the roles they might in designing the material world or health care they inhabit with their patients (Engebretson & Wardell, 1991; Greg-ory, 1993; Lenehan, 1991; Philip, 1987; Rebar, 1991; Stevens, 1994). Ac-cordingly, nursing offers a site to study opportunities and barriers to women's invention and participation in technology fields.

A Site to Study Women as Users of Technology

Nursing is an important empirical site for gender-technology studies also because nurses are a group primarily of women who interrupt the Western cultural association between technology and masculinity. Nurs-ing offers gender-technology scholars the opportunity to explore whether, and under what circumstances, this cultural association is largely ideological or empirical.

Although a constituency of nurses (at least since the mid-1970s) has viewed technology as an expression of male/medical culture that is an-tithetical to female/nursing culture (Allen & Hall 1988; Sandelowski, 1988; Ujhely, 1974), most nurses have readily incorporated technology into nursing practice and embraced technology as a means toward pro-fessional advancement and improved patient care. Indeed, nurses remain the primary "machine-body tenders" in health care (Fagerhaugh et al., 1987, pp. 81–82). Far from being technophobic or technically inept fe-males alienated from technological society, nurses have been eager, ac-tive, and competent users of complex technologies. Indeed, some feminists have criticized nurses (and women physicians) for this eager-ness, charging them with colluding with physicians in the deployment of technologies harmful to women, such as in-vitro fertilization (Wil-liams, 1989). Yet, nurses may use the technologies they share with phy-sicians and technicians differently and more humanely (Jones & Alexander, 1993; Ray, 1987). Whether such differences exist and whether they are due to gender, professional socialization, technical training, or other factors are questions that can be answered by selecting nursing as the site for study.

A Site to Study Gender, Culture, and Transfer
of Technology

Nursing also provides an important venue to study the transfer of technology between two "cultures": the cultures of medicine and nursing. With the nineteenth-century advent of diagnostic instrumentation (such as the clinical thermometer, the stethoscope, and the sphygmo-manometer) in medical practice, nurses assumed new functions as "machine tenders and measurement takers" (Howell, 1988, p. x). These functions eventually came to "dominate the interior life of hospitals and the work day of nurses" (Lynaugh & Fagin, 1988, p. 185). Lacking both the time and the inclination to make full use of these devices in practice, physicians increasingly ceded much of the work (even if not the authority over the work) associated with this new instrumentation to nurses and technicians. Full use of the mercury thermometer, for example, required frequent use of the device and recording of temperature over a 24-hour period to discern patterns of disease and response to treatment.

Moreover, devices such as the thermometer permitted the work to be segmented into tasks that could be delegated to others. When the thermometer was first introduced into practice in the mid-nineteenth century, physicians were concerned whether nurses or family members could be entrusted with its use. Only physicians were deemed capable of interpreting the meaning of a recorded temperature and initiating clinical action on the basis of that interpretation. Indeed, an argument offered for why it might be acceptable to delegate the discrete tasks of taking and recording the temperature to nurses was that they would not be distracted by everything physicians knew about the science of clinical thermometry (Reiser, 1993; Wunderlich, 1871). Yet, early on, nurses were taught to interpret temperature readings.

The example of the thermometer suggests that new medical technologies permitted tasks to be segmented in ways that both degraded and created opportunities for the advancement of nursing practice. Tasks appeared to be segmented into "physical" and "judgmental" components (Hershey, 1966), with physicians playing the central role in defining the scope of both medical and nursing practice. When a technique was deemed appropriate only for physicians to perform, it was valorized as a complex skill. Once the technique passed to nursing, it was degraded as a simple skill and feminized as a nursing, as opposed to a medical, activity (O'Hara, 1989). In his influential manual of medical thermometry, Wunderlich (1871) had trivialized the work of non-physician attendants to the sick, by declaring that the "mere reading of temperature degrees helps diagnosis no more than dispensing does therapeusis" (p. 75). Taking, reading, and recording the temperature (and the cleaning and maintenance thermometers required) were regarded as less complex than interpreting the temperature, and the people carrying out these former tasks were viewed as having less capabilities than those who engaged in the latter task.

Although the delegation to nurses of skills that physicians considered easy enough for a nurse to do may have degraded nursing work, it also appears to have given nurses the opportunity to become skilled in the tasks not officially delegated to them. To this day, nurses perform services rhetorically promoted, legally recognized, and financially rewarded as *medical* services.

Another interesting opportunity for studying gender and the transfer of technology between medicine and nursing concerns ostensibly gender-neutral needle therapies. As I summarized elsewhere (Sandelowski, 1997a), prior to the 1940s, the main bodily entries that American nurses were permitted involved nutrition and feeding and the elimination of waste. Nurses instilled and removed air and gases, fluids and substances for various cleaning, nutritional, and other therapeutic purposes. They used inhalers and tents for various kinds of respiratory and oxygen therapies, rubber or glass tubing to suction, gavage, lavage, administer enemas, douche, irrigate, and catheterize. These kinds of bodily entries emphasized the viscerality and literal "dirty work" of everyday nursing practice. Although nurses gave hypodermic injections in the nineteenth century and hypodermoclysis injections in the early twentieth century (both involving insertion of needles in tissue just beneath the skin), it was well into the 1930s before the intramuscular injection was conceived as appropriate for a nurse to administer. Intravenous instillation of substances and the removal of blood remained controversial as nursing functions until well into the 1960s. Many activities that involved deep piercing of the body with a needle or other implements were seen as exclusively in the physician's domain, with nurses assigned assistive function. Such bodily penetrations were arguably *cleaner* than the kind entailed in administering enemas, and they call into question the kinds of *penetrating body work* considered appropriate for nurses and physicians.

Yet, assistance with these cleaner procedures still meant doing everything involved in the procedure except the discrete act of piercing the skin. Whether assisting physicians to perform a paracentesis, lumbar puncture, or surgery, nurses were expected to have the knowledge to prepare and set up the equipment, prepare the patient and the room, and care for the patient and equipment after the procedure, which included watching for untoward treatment effects and cleaning up. This kind of division of labor, where nurses did everything-but (in the case of needle therapies, everything but the very discrete act of penetration), often characterized how nurses and physicians shared the same technologies. Moreover, this division of labor often defined the process by which the use of the same technologies was apparently controlled to maintain a line between medicine and nursing.

With a gender-technology studies slant, the history of delegation of medical technology to nurses can be reconceptualized as the story of how skill has become not an "objectively identifiable quality" but, rather, an "ideological category" over which women (here, nurses) were (and continue to be) "denied the rights of contestation" (Gill & Grint, 1995, p. 9). Moreover, the transfer of technology between historically male and female subcultures can be explored for the problems such transfers often entail. That is, what is technology; but also values, norms, and practices that may be in conflict with the receiving culture. Receiving cultures may, in turn, alter technologies to the extent that they are no longer the same as the technology transferred. Technologies are what they are, to a large extent, because of what they became in various use-contexts (Ihde, 1990). Nursing offers gender-technology scholars a site to study ostensibly the same technology in various gender contexts.

CONCLUSION

A scholarly rapprochement between nursing and gender-technology studies promises to advance the theoretical development and social agendas of both fields. I have offered here only the broad outlines of such a link, and the research agenda enabled by forging this link. A foray into gender-technology studies may offer nurses and nursing the space, visibility, and voice that still elude them, and a way of understanding and enabling nursing practice. A foray into nursing may offer gender-technology scholars (who may also be nursing scholars) the most fruitful site yet for the exploration of the mutual (re)constitution of gender and technology.

ACKNOWLEDGMENT

I am indebted to Joan Lynaugh for pointing out the importance, but lack of "sexiness" as an object of inquiry, of the bed in nursing history.

REFERENCES

Allen, D. G., Allman, K. M., & Powers, P. (1991). Feminist nursing research without gender. *Advances in Nursing Science, 13*, 49–58.
Allen, J. D., & Hall, B. A. (1988). Challenging the focus on technology: A critique of the medical model. *Advances in Nursing Science, 10*, 22–33.
Annandale, E., & Clark, J. (1996). What is gender? Feminist theory and the sociology of human reproduction. *Sociology of Health & Illness, 18*, 17–44.
Apple, R. D. (1987). *Mothers & medicine: A social history of infant feeding, 1890–1950*. Madison: University of Wisconsin Press.
Baer, E. (1991, February 19). The feminist disdain for nursing. *New York Times*.
Baker, J. P. (1996). *The machine in the nursery: Incubator technology and the origins of newborn intensive care*. Baltimore, MD: Johns Hopkins University Press.
Bankert, M. (1989). *Watchful care: A history of America's nurse anesthetists*. New York: Continuum.

Berg, A. J., & Lie, M. (1995). Feminism and constructivism: Do artifacts have gender? *Science, Technology, & Human Values, 20,* 332–351.

Bledstein, B. J. (1976). *The culture of professionalism: The middle class and the development of higher education in America.* New York: W. W. Norton.

Bottorff, J. L. (1991). Nursing: A practical science of caring. *Advances in Nursing Science, 14,* 26–39.

Cowan, R. S. (1983). *More work for mother: The ironies of household technology from the open hearth to the microwave.* New York: Basic Books.

Douglas, D. M. (1982). The machine in the parlor: A dialectical analysis of the sewing machine. *Journal of American Culture, 5,* 20–30.

Engebretson, J., & Wardell, D. (1991). Technology development: Protecting our ideas. *MCN: American Journal of Maternal-Child Nursing, 16,* 191–195.

Fagerhaugh, S. Y., Strauss, A., Suczek, B., & Wiener, C. (1987). *Hazards in hospital care: Ensuring patient safety.* San Francisco: Jossey-Bass.

Fagin, C. (1994). Women and nursing, today and tomorrow. In E. Friedman (Ed.), *An unfinished revolution: Women and health care in America* (pp. 159–176). New York: United Hospital Fund of New York.

Fairman, J. (1992). Watchful vigilance: Nursing care, technology, and the development of intensive care units. *Nursing Research, 41,* 56–60.

Faulkner, W., & Arnold, E. (Eds.). (1985). *Smothered by invention: Technology in women's lives.* London: Pluto.

Ferguson, E. S. (1977). The mind's eye: Nonverbal thought in technology. *Science, 197,* 827–836.

Gill, R., & Grint, K. (1995). The gender-technology relation: Contemporary theory and research. In K. Grint & R. Gill (Eds.), *The gender-technology relation: Contemporary theory and research* (pp. 1–28). London: Taylor and Francis.

Gordon, L. (1991). On "difference." *Genders, 10,* 91–111.

Gordon, S. (1991). *Prisoners of men's dreams: Striking out for a new feminine future.* Boston: Little, Brown.

Gregory, M. M. (1993). Technology in critical care unit design. *Critical Care Nursing Quarterly, 16,* 3.

Griffith, H. M., & Robinson, K. R. (1992). Survey of the degree to which critical care nurses are performing current procedural terminology-coded services. *American Journal of Critical Care, 1,* 91–95.

Grint, K., & Gill, R. (1995). *The gender-technology relation: Contemporary theory and research.* London: Taylor and Francis.

Grint, K., & Woolgar, S. (1995). On some failures of nerve in constructivist and feminist analyses of technology. *Science, Technology, & Human Values, 20,* 286–310.

Harmer, B. (1922). *Textbook of the principles and practice of nursing* (p. 33). New York: Macmillan.

Harney, M. (1993). Computation and gender. *Research in Philosophy and Technology, 13,* 57–71.

Harris, R. M. (1966). Symposium on the nurse and the new machinery (foreword). *Nursing Clinics of North America, 1,* 535–536.

Hershey, N. (1966). Scope of nursing practice. *American Journal of Nursing, 66,* 117–120.

Hoffart, N. (1989). Nephrology nursing, 1915–1970: A historical study of the integration of technology and care. *American Nurses' Nephrology Association Journal, 16,* 169–178.

Howell, J. D. (Ed.). (1988). *Technology and American medical practice, 1880–1930: Anthology of sources.* New York: Garland.

Hynes, P. H. (Ed.). (1991). *Reconstructing Babylon: Essays on women and technology.* Bloomington: Indiana University Press.

Ihde, D. (1979). *Technics and praxis.* Dordrecht, Netherlands: D. Reidel.

Ihde, D. (1990). *Technology and the lifeworld: From garden to earth.* Bloomington: Indiana University Press.

Jacox, A. (1992). Health care technology and its assessment: Where nursing fits in. In L. H. Aiken & C. M. Fagin (Eds.), *Charting nursing's future: Agenda for the 1990s* (pp. 70–84). Philadelphia: J. B. Lippincott.

Johnson, J. L. (1991). Nursing science: Basic, applied, or practical? Implications for the art of nursing. *Advances in Nursing Science, 14,* 7–16.

Jones, C. B., & Alexander, J. W. (1993). The technology of caring: A synthesis of technology and caring for nursing administration. *Nursing Administration Quarterly, 17,* 11–20.

Kim, H. S. (1994). Practice theories in nursing and a science of nursing practice. *Scholarly Inquiry for Nursing Practice, 8,* 145–166.

Kirkup, G., & Keller, L. S. (1992). *Inventing women: Science, technology and gender.* Cambridge: Polity Press.

Koenig, B. A. (1988). The technological imperative in nursing practice: The social creation of a "routine" treatment. In M. Lock & D. Gordon (Eds.), *Biomedicine examined* (pp. 465–496). Dordrecht, Netherlands: Kluwer Academic Publishers.

Lawler, J. (1991). *Behind the screens: Nursing, somology, and the problem of the body.* Melbourne, Australia: Churchill Livingstone.

Lenehan, G. P. (1991). Emergency nurses: Knowledgeable participants in the medical equipment arena (editorial). *Journal of Emergency Nursing, 17,* 61–62.

Lynaugh, J. (1988). Narrow passageways: Nurses and physicians in conflict and concert since 1875. In N. M. King, L. R. Churchill, & A. W. Cross (Eds.), *The physician as captain of the ship: A critical reappraisal* (pp. 23–37). Dordrecht, Netherlands: D. Reidel.

Lynaugh, J. (1989). Riding the yo-yo: The worth and work of nursing in the 20th century. *Transactions & Studies of the College of Physicians of Philadelphia, 11,* 201–217.

Lynaugh, J. (1994). Women and nursing: A historical perspective. In E. Friedman (Ed.), *An unfinished revolution: Women and health care in America* (pp. 143–163). New York: United Hospital Fund of New York.

Lynaugh, J. E., & Fagin, C. M. (1988). Nursing comes of age. *Image: Journal of Nursing Scholarship, 20,* 184–190.

McGaw, J. A. (1982). Women and the history of American technology. *Signs: Journal of Women in Culture and Society, 7,* 798–828.

Melosh, B. (1982). *The physician's hand: Work culture and conflict in American nursing.* Philadelphia: Temple University Press.

O'Hara, L. (1989). The operating theater as degradation ritual: A student nurse's view. *Science as Culture, 6,* 78–103.

Parker, J., & Gardner, G. (1992). The silence and silencing of the nurse's voice: A reading of patient progress notes. *Australian Journal of Advanced Nursing, 9*, 3–9.

Perry, R. (Ed.). (1990). From hard drive to software: Gender, computers, and difference (special issue). *Signs: Journal of Women in Culture and Society, 16*, 1.

Philip, J. (1987). The nurse as designer: Product development. *Nursing, 3*, 831–833.

Ratcliff, K. S. (Ed.). (1989). *Healing technology: Feminist perspectives.* Ann Arbor: University of Michigan Press.

Ray, M. A. (1987). Technological caring: A new model in critical care. *Dimensions of Critical Care Nursing, 6*, 166–173.

Rebar, L. A. (1991). The nurse as inventor: Obtain a patent and benefit from your ideas. *AORN Journal, 53*, 468–478.

Reiser, S. J. (1993). Technology and the use of the senses in twentieth-century medicine. In W. F. Bynum & R. Porter (Eds.), *Medicine and the five senses* (pp. 262–323). Cambridge: Cambridge University Press.

Reverby, S. M. (1989). A legitimate relationship: Nursing, hospitals, and science in the twentieth century. In D. E. Long & J. Golden (Eds.), *The American general hospital: Communities and social contexts* (pp. 135–156). Ithaca, NY: Cornell University Press.

Roberts, J. I., & Group, T. M. (1995). *Feminism and nursing: An historical perspective on power, status, and political activism in the nursing profession.* Westport, CT: Praeger.

Rosenberg, C. E. (1987). *The care of strangers: The rise of America's hospital system.* New York: Basic Books.

Rothschild, J. (Ed.). (1983). *Machina ex dea: Feminist perspectives on technology.* New York: Pergamon Press.

Rothschild, J. (1988). *Teaching technology from a feminist perspective.* New York: Pergamon Press.

Sandelowski, M. A. (1988). A case of conflicting paradigms: Nursing and reproductive technology. *Advances in Nursing Science, 10*, 35–45.

Sandelowski, M. (1997a). Knowing and forgetting: The challenge of technology for a reflexive practice science of nursing. In S. Thorne & J. Hayes (Eds.), *Clinical knowledge and praxis in nursing.* Thousand Oaks, CA: Sage.

Sandelowski, M. (1997b). "Making the best of things": Technology in American nursing, 1870–1940. *Nursing History Review, 5*, 3–22.

Sandelowski, M. (1997c). (Ir)Reconcilable differences? The debate concerning nursing and technology. *Image: Journal of Nursing Scholarship, 29*, 169–174.

Smith, M. R. (1932). What are we doing to improve nursing practice, II: Through improvement of nursing methods. *American Journal of Nursing 32*, 685–688.

Spallone, P., & Steinberg, D. L. (Eds.). (1987). *Made to order: The myth of reproductive and genetic progress.* Oxford: Pergamon Press.

Stanley, A. (1995). *Mothers and daughters of invention: Notes for a revised history of technology.* New Brunswick, NJ: Rutgers University Press.

Stanworth, M. (Ed.). (1987). *Reproductive technologies: Gender, motherhood and medicine.* Minneapolis: University of Minnesota Press.

Stevens, K. R. (1994). Patents and the nurse scholar, Part I: The basic philosophy of intellectual property. *Reflections, 20,* 36–38.

Strauss, A., Fagerhaugh, S., Suczek, B., & Wiener, C. (1982). Sentimental work in the technologized hospital. *Sociology of Health & Illness, 4,* 254–277.

Traweek, S. (1993). An introduction to cultural and social studies of sciences and technologies. *Culture, Medicine and Psychiatry, 17,* 3–25.

Trescott, M. M. (Ed.). (1979). *Dynamos and virgins revisited: Women and technological change in history.* Metuchen, NJ: Scarecrow Press.

Ujhely, G. B. (1974). Current technological advances and the nurse-patient relationship. *Journal of New York State Nurses' Association, 5,* 25–28.

Wajcman, J. (1991). *Feminism confronts technology.* University Park: Pennsylvania State University Press.

Walker, K. (1994). Confronting "reality": Nursing, science and the micropolitics of representation. *Nursing Inquiry, 1,* 46–56.

West, C., & Zimmerman, D. H. (1987). Doing gender. *Gender & Society, 1,* 125–151.

Williams, L. S. (1989). The overlooked role of women professionals in the provision of in vitro fertilization. *Resources for Feminist Research, 18,* 80–82.

Wolf, Z. R. (1986). Nurses' work: The sacred and the profane. *Holistic Nursing Practice, 1,* 29–35.

Wolf, Z. R. (1989). Uncovering the hidden work of nursing. *Nursing & Health Care, 10,* 463–467.

Woolgar, S. (Ed.). (1995). Feminist and constructivist perspectives on new technology (special issue). *Science, Technology, & Human Values, 20,* 3.

Wunderlich, C. A. (1871). *On the temperature in diseases: A manual of medical thermometry* (W. B. Woodman, Trans.). London: New Sydenham Society.

Zalumas, J. (1995). *Caring in crisis: An oral history of critical care nursing.* Philadelphia: University of Pennsylvania Press.

Chapter 17

Problem-Based Learning and Technology: A Caring Pedagogy in Nursing

Constance M. Baker

INTRODUCTION

The knowledge explosion, technology, economics, and demographics have revolutionized health care delivery. The dramatic transformation of health care delivery necessitates a dramatic transformation in nursing education. The emerging managed care environment and the demand for evidence-based practice and data-driven outcomes require nurses who can engage in critical thinking and clinical reasoning. Indeed, skills in "critical thinking and critical judgment" are the first priority in the American Association of Colleges of Nursing's (AACN) latest Position Statement on nursing education (AACN, 1999). Nursing faculty are challenged to evaluate the current evolution of a market-driven health care delivery system, anticipate the consolidated network systems of the future, and attend to the curriculum consequences of such statements as Pew's "Twenty-one Competencies for the 21st Century" (Bellack & O'Neil, 2000).

Extraordinary gains in communication and information technology are influencing faculties' philosophy of teaching and learning, program delivery practices, and students' expectations (Diekelmann, Schuster, & Nosek, 1998). Both communication technology (electronic mail, listserv, electronic conferencing systems, chat rooms, coffee houses) and information technology (World Wide Web, search engines, online journals, web-based courses) are being used to deliver academic courses. Comprehensive efforts to assess the outcomes of web-based courses are underway, focusing on the interaction of the technology, educational practices, faculty support, and learner support (Billings, 2000). National higher education organizations are participating in the dialogue about the complex challenges and the rewards of the new technologies (*Academe*, 1999; *Change*, 1999).

Educators in the health professions are challenged to design student learning opportunities related to computer technologies and information science. Health professionals are facing escalating information management challenges in clinical practice as computer technology permeates all aspects of patient care (Ball et al., 2000). Professional organizations and accrediting bodies have issued statements regarding preparation of contemporary nurses in computer technology (AACN, 1999; IMIA, 1999). Specifically, nurses must be able to use the information systems operating in their places of employment. Employers assume nurses have the ability to use computer technology and electronic networks for communication with other professionals. Nurses should be able to search, retrieve, and organize information from a variety of computerized information sources. Nurses need to be able to seek information for decision making through expert systems and knowledge databases in patient care. The professional literature has many case studies of schools of nursing redesigning their curricula to include more instruction in computer technology and information science (Travis & Brennan, 1998).

The stage for redesigning nursing education has been set by the outcomes of nursing's ongoing "curriculum revolution": familiarity with humanistic existentialism, centrality of caring concepts, primacy of teacher-student relationship, increased service learning and social responsibility, and critical reflection (Metcalfe, 1998; Tanner, 1990). Descriptions of nursing education's future include demands of both the clinical practice settings and the university environments (Heller, Oros, & Durney-Crowley, 2000; Lindeman, 2000). A persistent theme throughout this literature is the need for meaningful faculty-student relationships within communities of caring.

An analysis of four prominent, conceptual perspectives on caring in nursing concludes that they are grounded in humanism and reflect nursing's dual components: attitudes and activities (McCance, McKenna, & Boore, 1999). A fifth perspective, derived from phenomenological investigations, defines caring as "a nurturing way of relating to a valued other toward whom one has a personal sense of commitment and responsibility" (Swanson, 1991, p. 162). Caring involves five therapeutic processes. These are maintaining belief (in the other's potential to get through an event or transition and face a meaningful future), knowing (informed striving to understand the other's experience), being with (emotionally present), doing for (as the other would do for self if she had the knowledge or capability), and enabling (facilitating resolution by validating, informing) (Swanson, 1993). Thus, caring involves deliberate, rational, and knowledgeable acts of assisting another's goal achievement, a balance between scientific knowledge and humanistic practice behaviors (Komorita, Doehring, & Hirchert, 1991).

When applied to nursing education, faculty behaviors include creating a learner-focused curriculum, developing a trusting partnership with students, anticipating student needs in seeking knowledge, being accessible to students, explaining and facilitating collaborative learning, supporting students' efforts to resolve cognitive dissonance, and modeling critical reflection. One educational strategy to prepare reflective nurse clinicians who engage in critical thinking and clinical reasoning is problem-based learning (PBL), a discovery method of teaching which was promoted in the 1930s and has been implemented in the health science professions since the 1970s (Baker, 2000b).

THE NATURE OF PROBLEM-BASED LEARNING

Problem-based learning is an educational approach characterized by the use of a "real-life" problem as the context for a group of students to learn clinical reasoning skills and acquire knowledge about the problem (Barrows & Tamblyn, 1980). Problem-based learning has several fundamental and unique characteristics: the problem, small group of students, tutor-facilitator, a goal-oriented multisession unit, learning objectives, self-directed learning time, concept mapping, and evaluation (DeGoeij, 1997). Evaluation is an integral part of each problem discussion meeting, culminating at the final session with evaluation of the case, the learning resources, the tutor-facilitator, the group, and the student.

Problem-based learning differs from traditional pedagogies in several key dimensions: focus is on student-centered learning, teacher is a coach and tutor, students actively seek knowledge in a group-centered environment, learning activity is problem-solving, and the outcomes include self-directed learning and clinical reasoning skills. Problem-based learning differs from the case method in two key ways: the problem is presented first, before students have learned basic knowledge; and the problem is presented in stages, stimulating the student to seek additional information. The underlying assumptions derived from cognitive psychology are:

- students use prior knowledge to understand and structure new information
- transfer of learning is more likely to occur when the problems resemble real-life situations
- knowledge retention is enhanced through such elaboration activities as peer discussion, questioning, and critiquing (Norman & Schmidt, 1992).

Problem-based learning is consistent with constructivism, the philosophical view that knowledge is not absolute, but is "constructed" by the learner based on previous knowledge and worldview. Three primary constructivist principles reflected in problem-based learning are that (1) understanding comes from interaction with the environment, (2) cognitive conflict stimulates learning, and (3) knowledge evolves through social negotiation and evaluation of the viability of individual understandings (Savery & Duffy, 1995). Thus, problem-based learning creates the opportunity for the learner to find knowledge for oneself, to contrast one's understanding of that knowledge with others' understanding, and to refine or restructure knowledge as more relevant experience is gained (Savin-Baden, 1997; Stinson & Milter, 1996).

Worldwide Diffusion

Problem-based learning has been used in medical schools for 30 years; in some Canadian, Australian, and British nursing schools for nearly 10 years; and has recently spread into most health sciences and other disciplines (Baker, 2000a). In nursing, McMaster University School of Nursing pioneered problem-based learning curricula and has sustained its evolution with annual summer workshops that support nursing faculty development in the method. The McMaster model of problem-based learning has been adopted in several schools in Australia and the United Kingdom. Professional literature reveals that nursing schools are using problem-based learning in selected courses in South Africa, China, Japan, and Thailand. Seven U.S. nursing schools are represented in the problem-based learning literature: five use PBL in community health nursing, one uses PBL in nursing administration, and one describes multicultural students' experience with problem-based learning (Baker, 2000b). Each of these U.S. nursing education programs is located in a university where the medical school has implemented PBL. Recently, the Pew Charitable Trust funded Stanford University to use PBL to redesign the undergraduate curriculum in arts and sciences, business, education, nursing, and pharmacy. This demonstration project includes a PBL research center to assess the entire PBL effort and disseminate the research findings (www.stanford.edu/pbl).

Preparation

A major implementation issue is the preparation of faculty and students for a new philosophy of teaching and learning (Woods, 1994). Faculties need support to move from lecture-based traditional courses and standard textbooks to the tutor-coach role in problem-based courses and integrating materials from several disciplines. Numerous authors allude to faculty anxiety in moving from "the sage on the stage" to the "guide at the side" (Stinson & Milter, 1996). Faculties usually need assistance to orient students to the new expectations of active and collaborative learning, and support when students complain about the requirements of active participation. Students need instruction to refine their skills in self-directed learning, group process, problem solving, self-assessment, and peer review (Modell, 1996). Information-seeking skills and library supports are critical to success and may be part of student orientation or an introductory course. Student anxiety has been interpreted as a necessary motivating force to stimulate students' "need to know" and their desire to actively pursue self-directed learning activities. Students need support in learning how to cope with the disequilibrium they experience when they are expected to move from a passive learning environment and relinquish previously successful academic behaviors to an active learning environment and assume responsibility for their own learning (Savin-Baden, 1997; Stinson & Milter, 1996).

Process

The classic problem-based learning unit usually consists of three to five meetings: a problem presentation meeting, problem discussion meetings, and an evaluation session. In the problem presentation meeting students approach the problem by organizing information in the initial scenario into three categories: facts, hypotheses, and learning issues. A fact is a piece of given information, a hypothesis is a hunch or proposed explanation of the problem, and a learning issue is information that is needed to solve the problem (Stanhope & Sebastian, 1999).

After students seek the needed information, a second problem discussion meeting is convened in which students share their new knowledge, analyze the information relative to learning issues and the hypotheses, create concept maps, critique learning resources, and assess reasoning processes used in specifying hypotheses and learning issues (Andrews & Jones, 1996). A second section of the scenario is distributed which relaunches the process of organizing information, restructuring facts, hypotheses, and learning issues, and seeking additional information. In the final meeting, after the problem is solved and the concepts are mapped, the learning objectives are used as the basis for evaluation of the students' learning, the group's competence, and the facilitator's capability.

Participants

The people involved in the problem-based learning unit include the students, the teacher-facilitator, and human learning resources. The ideal size of a group is six to nine students, to ensure that all students participate in problem analysis (Barrows & Tamblyn, 1980). The group needs a recorder and may designate another student to lead the case discussion.

Students' self-directed learning time is the period between the problem presentation and problem discussion meetings. Individual students or small groups seek information to satisfy the identified learning issues and then may restructure the problem based on new knowledge. Students seek information from print, electronic, and multimedia resources and human resources. Information-seeking skills and library support are critical to success and are usually included in student orientation (Schilling et al., 1995; Woods, 1994).

The tutor-facilitator has a very active coaching role in monitoring verbal and non-verbal interactions to facilitate group process and enhance learning (Frost, 1996). The primary teaching strategy is posing questions (Cooke & Donovan, 1998). The tutor has five key responsibilities. These include:

- ask meta-cognitive questions to ensure that the problem is examined in sufficient depth and breadth,
- expand each student's interpretative thinking skills by calling on each student to summarize the case,
- involve non-participating students by asking direct questions,
- regulate domineering students by asking mitigating questions,
- monitor class time by asking questions of intent.

Several people are considered learning resources, beginning with the librarian, who is the key in PBL. Professional experts and clients may also provide information for students' inquiry. Faculty specify the learning objectives for each problem and distribute them near the end of the problem presentation session, to avoid interfering with the student-generated learning issues. The learning objectives provide one perspective for evaluation at the conclusion of the problem analysis. Both formative and summative evaluations are used to assess performances of the student (Stanhope & Sebastian, 1999), the group, and the tutor (Hay, 1997); the PBL process (Chaves, Chaves, & Lantz, 1998), and the learning resources. In addition to the traditional testing methods, individual student evaluation in problem-based learning may include journals, self-evaluations, and the "triple jump," a culminating exercise designed for each student to individually demonstrate to the faculty the problem-based learning process with his/her own case (O'Neill, 1998).

Outcomes

Expected outcomes of the problem-based learning method are: develops clinical reasoning, structures knowledge in real life contexts, motivates learning, and develops self-learning skills (Barrows, 1998).

However, different disciplines have modified the original conceptualization of PBL so synthesizing educational outcomes research is extremely difficult. A wide range of study designs is used in assessing outcomes, ranging from case studies to experimental designs. Some of the research articles report evaluation of entire curricula and other articles report assessment of a single course (Boud & Feletti, 1997).

Medicine leads other disciplines with well over 200 articles reporting quantitative evaluation research on problem-based learning (Albanese & Mitchell, 1993; Vernon & Blake, 1993). A summary of the experimental evidence on the psychological basis of some of the problem-based learning outcomes concludes that a problem-based curriculum enhances transfer of concepts to new problems and clinical applications, fosters increased retention of knowledge, increases intrinsic interest in the subject, and strengthens self-directed learning skills (Norman & Schmidt, 1992). Students in problem-based learning curricula exceeded traditional students in clinical knowledge tests, clinical performance, and satisfaction with academic program. Faculty satisfaction is higher in schools with problem-based curricula and they especially enjoy the curricular aspects of the academic process (Norman & Schmidt, 1992).

Evaluation research of problem-based learning in nursing education tends to be qualitative and course-based, with a range of outcomes. In two case studies, nursing students did not acquire the expected level of knowledge, in part related to unrealistic scenarios, physical constraints, and inadequate tutor preparation (Andrews & Jones, 1996; Frost, 1996). Both formative and summative evaluations have been positive in a series of master's courses in community health nursing (Stanhope & Sebastian, 1999). In an ethnographic study of 12 graduates from a problem-based curriculum, the graduates described their transition from student to staff nurse, identified personal characteristics which distinguished them from graduates of traditional curricula, and spoke to their responsibility for lifelong learning and becoming a change-agent (Biley & Smith, 1998). Another report from a problem-based curriculum is a study of predictors of success on the state board examination at the McMaster University School of Nursing (Carpio, O'Mara, & Hezekiah, 1996). More evaluation studies are expected as PBL becomes more widespread in nursing education programs and nurse researchers extend the qualitative data to large, quantitative studies. Evaluation of PBL methods is an important area in the scholarship of teaching.

USING TECHNOLOGY TO IMPLEMENT PBL

Like most institutions of higher education in the United States, Indiana University has a very sophisticated computer-supported instructional environment. The School of Nursing offers nearly one-third of the undergraduate and master's programs through asynchronous Internet courses. Many faculty in the other courses integrate online activities into traditional classroom formats. Faculty in Nursing Administration recently launched a redesigned master's program using PBL. The cases are delivered via the executive format of one weekend a month with asynchronous computer conferencing between weekends to continue the study of case-related learning issues and group projects.

This weekend delivery method allows for problem presentation in a traditional, face-to-face seminar, but computer technology can be used in every step of the PBL process. In fact, business faculty at Ohio University offer the entire Master's of Business Administration (M.B.A.) online, using PBL and computer technology (Stinson & Milter, 1996). When the problem scenario is presented online, students are able to prepare in advance by gleaning initial information from a computer-based case (Bresnitz, 1996). The students' self-directed study includes using the World Wide Web to access data about learning issues from professional organizations, governmental agencies, libraries, and other stakeholders involved in the subject of the learning issue. Students present their synthesized data reports through online electronic communication and the other students in the course critique the computer entries, determine whether or not their PBL hypotheses have been supported, and may reframe the learning issue. Concept mapping can be launched on the Internet by differentiating definitions, linking key characteristics, and applying information to hypothesis testing. Students can initiate their own learning synthesis in their computer entries with each other, and faculty can stimulate the process by posing meta-cognitive questions on the computer. Web-based evaluation tools are being applied to all stakeholders in a PBL case: individual student, student peers, and tutors (Chaves, Chaves, & Lantz, 1998). Efforts are underway to assess students' critical thinking behaviors in their web-based discourse. Course evaluations can also be conducted on the computer.

Computer technology is beginning to be applied in generating problem-based learning cases and simulations, developing electronic study guides, creating computer-based (virtual) student groups, and implementing evaluation procedures. Curriculum development and management is being enhanced with specially designed computer tools (Field & Sefton, 1998). Computer simulations are being used as a research tool to document how students learn (Rendas, Pinto, & Gamboa, 1999).

A CARING PEDAGOGY FOR NURSING

Nursing faculty recognize their responsibility to prepare nurses who are critical thinkers and technologically proficient. Nurses are challenged to combine their scientific knowledge with a humanistic approach to their clients. Problem-based learning promises to produce knowledgeable critical thinking graduates who genuinely care for and about their patients (Bechtel & Davidhizar, 1999; Bechtel, Davidhizar, & Bradshaw, 1999; Heliker, 1994).

The learner-centered nature of problem-based learning forces faculty to address four aspects of learning: basic cognitive and meta-cognitive factors, motivational and affective factors, social and developmental factors, and individual differences in learning (Bonk & King, 1998). Faculty must consider how best to guide thinking, sustain motivation, foster social interaction, and maximize differences. The caring exhibited by faculty facilitating problem-based learning is consistent with the definition of caring as "a nurturing way of relating to a valued other toward whom one has a personal sense of commitment and responsibility" (Swanson, 1991, p. 162). A learning community created in an academic course structured by PBL is a caring community. Self-directed searching for new knowledge and collaborative problem solving within a PBL teacher–student partnership leads to mutual respect and genuine caring. Presumably, if students experience genuine caring in their educational process, they will carry this learning into their clinical practice.

The dimensions of learner experiences in PBL courses have been described in a model focused on three stances: personal, pedagogical, and interactional (Savin-Baden, 1997). The personal stance includes the means by which students discover, define, and place themselves within the PBL environment. The pedagogical stance refers to how students see themselves as learners and includes their prior learning experiences, their relationships between the self and the course content, and their personal reflections on the interaction of these aspects and the requisite disjunctions and paradoxes. The interactional stance refers to how learners interact with others in the PBL course environment and how they construct meaning in relation to one another. Caring faculty have unique opportunities in each of these three learner stances to demonstrate their beliefs that students have potential to learn, their awareness of students' striving efforts, their emotional presence in the teacher–student partnership, and their teaching and facilitation skills. Thus, faculty caring is demonstrated in PBL courses through deliberate, rational, and knowledgeable acts of assisting students' goal achievements, a balance between scientific knowledge and humanistic teacher behaviors.

The excellent potential of problem-based learning to prepare caring professional nurses has been supported with ample research from other health disciplines and emerging research from nursing schools in Australia, Canada, the United Kingdom, and the United States. Any reluctance of nursing faculty to recognize this paradigm shift in education and to investigate the potential of problem-based learning requires the dean's visionary leadership in curriculum development and assessment.

In an information society demanding evidence-based practice, it is imperative that nurses be prepared to locate, critique, and apply the latest information to the care of their patients. Problem-based learning holds that promise for caring nurse educators.

REFERENCES

Academe: Bulletin of American Association of University Professors (1999). *85*(5), entire issue.

Albanese, M. A., & Mitchell, S. (1993). Problem-based learning: A review of literature on its outcomes and implementation issues. *Academic Medicine, 68*, 52–81.

American Association of Colleges of Nursing (AACN). (1999). Position statement: A vision of baccalaureate and graduate nursing education: The next decade. *Journal of Professional Nursing, 15*, 59–65.

Andrews, M., & Jones, P. R. (1996). Problem-based learning in an undergraduate nursing programme: A case study. *Journal of Advanced Nursing, 23*, 357–365.

Baker, C. M. (2000a). Using problem-based learning to redesign nursing administration masters programs. *Journal of Nursing Administration, 30*(1), 41–47.

Baker, C. M. (2000b). Problem-based learning for nursing: Integrating lessons from other disciplines with nursing experiences. *Journal of Professional Nursing, 16*(5), in press.

Ball, M. J., Hannah, K. J., Newbold, S. K., & Douglas, J. V. (Eds.). (2000). *Nursing informatics: Where caring and technology meet* (3rd ed.). New York: Springer-Verlag.

Barrows, H. S. (1998). The essentials of problem-based learning. *Journal of Dental Education 62*, 630–633.

Barrows, H. S., & Tamblyn, R. M. (1980). *Problem-based learning: An approach to medical education*. New York: Springer.

Bechtel, G. A., & Davidhizar, R. (1999). An innovative education strategy in a migrant farm community. *Nurse Educator, 24*(1), 23–24.

Bechtel, G. A., Davidhizar, R., & Bradshaw, M. J. (1999). Problem-based learning in a competency-based world. *Nurse Education Today, 19*(3), 182–187.

Bellack, J. P., & O'Neil, E. H. (2000). Recreating nursing practice for a new century. *Nursing and Health Care Perspectives, 21*(1), 14–21.

Biley, F. C., & Smith, K. L. (1998). "The buck stops here": Accepting responsibility for learning and actions after graduation from a problem-based learning nursing education curriculum. *Journal of Advanced Nursing, 27*, 1021–1029.

Billings, D. M. (2000). A framework for assessing outcomes and practices in web-based courses in nursing. *Journal of Nursing Education, 39*(2), 60–67.

Bonk, C. J., & King, K. S. (Eds.). (1998). *Electronic collaborators: Learner-centered technologies for literacy, apprenticeship, and discourse*. Mahwah, NJ: Lawrence Erlbaum.

Boud, D., & Feletti, G. I. (Eds.). (1997). *The challenge of problem-based learning* (2nd ed.). London: Kogan Page Ltd.

Bresnitz, E. A. (1996). Computer-based learning in PBL. *Academic Medicine, 71*(5), 540.

Carpio, B., O'Mara, L., & Hezekiah, J. (1996). Predictors of success on the Canadian Nurses Association testing service (CNATS) examination. *Canadian Journal of Nursing Research, 28,* 115–123.

Change: The Magazine of Higher Learning. (1999). *31*(2), entire issue.

Chaves, J. F., Chaves, J. A., & Lantz, M. S. (1998). The PBL-Evaluator: A web-based tool for assessment in tutorials. *Journal of Dental Education, 62,* 671–674.

Cooke, M., & Donovan, A. (1998). The nature of the problem: The intentional design of problems to facilitate different levels of student learning. *Nurse Education Today, 18,* 462–469.

DeGoeij, A. F. (1997). Problem-based learning: What is it? What is it not? What about the basic sciences? *Biochemical Society Transactions, 25,* 288–293.

Diekelmann, N., Schuster, R., & Nosek, C. (1998). Creating new pedagogies at the millenium: The common experiences of the University of Wisconsin–Madison teachers using distance education technologies. *Teaching with Technology Today* (Online journal). Available: http://www.uwsa.edu/olit/ttt/98.pdf.

Field, M. J., & Sefton, A. J. (1998). Computer-based management of content in planning a problem-based medical curriculum. *Medical Education, 32,* 163–171.

Frost, M. (1996). An analysis of the scope and value of problem-based learning in the education of health professionals. *Journal of Advanced Nursing, 24,* 1047–1053.

Hay, J. A. (1997). An investigation of a tutor evaluation scale for formative purposes in a problem-based learning curriculum. *American Journal of Occupational Therapy, 51,* 140–143.

Heliker, D. (1994). Meeting the challenge of the curriculum revolution: Problem-based learning in nursing education. *Journal of Nursing Education, 33*(1), 45–47.

Heller, B. R., Oros, M. T., & Durney-Crowley, J. (2000). The future of nursing: Ten trends to watch. *Nursing and Health Care Perspectives, 21*(1), 9–13.

International Medical Informatics Association (IMIA). (1999, October). IMIA Recommendations on Education in Health and Medical Informatics. Available: http://www.imia.org/wg1.

Komorita, N. I., Doehring, K. M., & Hirchert, P. W. (1991). Perceptions of caring by nurse educators. *Journal of Nursing Education, 30*(1), 23–29.

Lindeman, C. A. (2000). The future of nursing education. *Journal of Nursing Education, 39*(1), 5–12.

McCance, T. V., McKenna, H. P., & Boore, J.R.P. (1999). Caring: Theoretical perspectives of relevance to nursing. *Journal of Advanced Nursing, 30*(6), 1388–1395.

Metcalfe, S. E. (1998). Behaviorism to humanism: The case for philosophical transformations in nursing education. *NursingConnections, 11*(4), 41–46.

Modell, H. I. (1996). Preparing students to participate in an active learning environment. *American Journal of Physiology, 270,* S69–S77.

Norman, G. R., & Schmidt, H. G. (1992). The psychological basis of problem-based learning: A review of the evidence. *Academic Medicine, 67,* 557–565.

O'Neill, P. N. (1998). Assessment of students in a problem-based learning curriculum. *Journal of Dental Education, 62,* 640–643.

Rendas, A., Rosado Pinto, P., & Gamboa, T. (1999). A computer simulation designed for problem-based learning. *Medical Education, 33,* 047–054.

Savery, J. R., & Duffy, T. M. (1995). Problem-based learning: An instructional model and its constructivist framework. *Educational Technology, 35*(5), 31–37.

Savin-Baden, M. (1997). Problem-based learning, Part 2: Understanding learners stances. *British Journal of Occupational Therapy, 60*(12), 531–535.

Schilling, K., Ginn, D. S., Mickelson, P., & Roth, L. H. (1995). Integration of information-seeking skills and activities into a problem-based curriculum. *Bulletin of the Medical Association, 83,* 176–183.

Stanhope, M., & Sebastian, J. G. (1999). *Instructor's resources guide to accompany case studies in community health nursing practice: A problem-based learning approach.* St. Louis, MO: Mosby.

Stinson, J. E., & Milter, R. G. (1996). Problem-based learning in business education: Curriculum design and implementation issues. In L. Wilkerson & W. Gijslaers (Eds.), *New directions in teaching and learning in higher education* (pp. 33–42). San Francisco: Jossey-Bass.

Swanson, K. M. (1991). Empirical development of a middle range theory of caring. *Nursing Research, 40*(3), 161–166.

Swanson, K. M. (1993). Nursing as informed caring for the well-being of others. *Image: Journal of Nursing Scholarship, 25*(4), 352–357.

Tanner, C. A. (1990). Reflections on the curriculum revolution. *Journal of Nursing Education, 29*(7), 295–299.

Travis, L., & Brennan, P. F. (1998). Information science for the future: An innovative nursing informatics curriculum. *Journal of Nursing Education, 37*(4), 162–168.

Vernon, D. T., & Blake, R. L. (1993). Does problem-based learning work? A meta-analysis of evaluative research. *Academic Medicine, 68,* 550–563.

Woods, D. R. (1994). *Problem-based learning: How to gain the most from PBL.* Waterdown, Ontario: Woods.

Chapter 18

Telehealth Nursing: Challenging Caring in Nursing

Lore K. Wright, Suzanne Pursley-Crotteau, and Loretta Schlachta-Fairchild

VIGNETTE

Every Wednesday afternoon, cancer patient Morris Evans (fictitious name) walks into his living room with a fresh cup of coffee, turns on his TV, and settles comfortably into his easy chair—for a visit from his telenurse! At the scheduled 2:00 P.M. time, Morris's phone rings and he picks up a remote control and hits the start button. The familiar, friendly voice of Jane Foster (fictitious name), Oncology Clinical Nurse Specialist, floats from the TV set: "Good afternoon, Morris. Is this a good time for us to visit?" Morris hits the start button again to turn on the video and sees the smiling face of Jane. How wonderful to see Jane, from the comfort of his own living room! After assessing Morris's overall status and disposition, they discuss Morris's temperature, whether he is able to eat, and how his young children are reacting to his hair loss. Jane takes a look at Morris's intravenous catheter site over the camera to make sure there is no sign of infection, and she spends some time discussing details of the upcoming round of chemotherapy with Morris and his wife. After completing their discussion, Jane makes an appointment for the same time next week, and reminds Morris that in the interim, he can obtain assistance for any acute issues by calling the telehealth call center. Morris reports how comforting it is to know that help is merely a videophone call away, especially since he lives two hours from the nearest hospital or clinic.

INTRODUCTION

Telehealth is the use of technology to facilitate interactive communication between nurses, patients/clients, and other health care providers. This technology transports clinical practice over time and distance to provide care to various patient populations. With the promise of an improved health care delivery system, many skeptics discount the potential for increased access and convenience because of concerns over the perceived loss of caring through the use of technology. In order to reframe this perception and situate care as integral in the processes of telehealth technology, it is critical to review challenges to the concept of caring from nursing theory and Noddings' (1984) theory of caring. Furthermore, existential phenomenology, particularly the work of Heidegger (1962), and the phenomenological nursing literature on caring and technology are relevant.

Heidegger (1962) believed caring provided the meaning to existence. From Heidegger's perspective, technology is useful as a part of the meaningful relationships inseparable from caring. Two phenomenological studies of critical care nurses (Ray, 1987; Walters, 1995) focused on the use of technology in the provision of nursing care. Both authors supported the notion that technology becomes phenomenologically transparent for the nurses because they are not always aware of its existence. According to Walters (1995), "the nurses' attention is directed not at the individual piece of technology per se but at the work that the technology is intended to perform which becomes subsumed in the caring process" (p. 7).

Heidegger (1962) also addressed the issue of when technology does not work or fails to perform its function. Currently, technical problems with telehealth systems are still fairly common. Thus, when telehealth equipment fails, practitioners are in flux, and the ability to care through this technological medium is compromised. Considering these caring perspectives, we will address the following: (1) the history of telehealth nursing, (2) the consumers' perspective of telehealth, (3) challenges of telehealth and the implications for the caring relationship, and (4) the future of telehealth nursing.

HISTORY OF TELEHEALTH NURSING

The roots of telehealth nursing lie in the history of telemedicine. Telemedicine is defined as the practice of health care delivery, diagnosis, consultation, treatment, transfer of medical data, and education using interactive audio, visual, and data communications (Kansas Telemedicine, Policy Group, 1993). Telehealth is a broader term often interchanged equally with telemedicine, and encompasses the same elements of interactivity. Telenursing is the use of telehealth technology to deliver nursing care and conduct nursing practice (Sparks & Schlachta, 1997).

The field of telehealth is not new, although it is currently undergoing a rapid resurgence and growth (Grigsby & Kaehny, 1993). In the early 1960s and 1970s, the efficacy of telemedicine for long distance diagnosis, consultation, education, and patient care in the fields of telepsychiatry, teledermatology, and telecardiology was demonstrated (Dwyer, 1973; Gravenstein et al., 1974; Murphy et al., 1973). Thirty years ago, however, the fiscal incentive for widespread use of telemedicine did not exist. Health care expense was not an issue, computer technology was cumbersome and prohibitively expensive, and telecommunications were primitive (Bashur, 1994). In contrast, today's computers, with capabilities that far exceed those of 30 years ago, can be purchased for home use for under $1,500. Affordable computer technology with capabilities for satellite, fiber-optic, and telephone communications, and the fiscal impetus to reorganize the way health care is provided, has resulted in what is generally referred to as telehealth technology (Grigsby & Kaehny, 1993). Telehealth technology ranges from POTS (plain old telephone service) to satellites. In between lies a myriad of telecommunications opportunities for conveying clinical information, depending on the quality and clarity of video and audio required by the clinical use. The use of the Internet is also revolutionizing telehealth, since providers can interact with each other and with patients. Data downloads can occur from any computer and be sent to providers for analysis and monitoring. Experience shows that the most successful telemedicine projects are those that use the simplest and least expensive form of technology required for clinical application (Anonymous, 1994). A satellite or fiber-optic system is not necessary for every clinical application. Cost increases as clarity and speed of technology increases.

Telehealth nursing is also not new. There is documented evidence of the existence of telehealth nurses for more than 25 years. However, empirical evidence of the practice and perceptions of nurses in telehealth is severely limited. Early descriptions of telehealth programs in the 1970s and 1980s alluded to nurses actively participating in telehealth work. Few specifics were offered. Later studies began to report data from active participation of nurses and even telehealth nurse–impacted patient outcomes.

The earliest reference to the role of a telehealth nurse was by Quinn (1974). She described her role as a nurse in a hospital-based telehealth center where she assumed the roles of technician, scheduler, patient educator, staff educator, coordinator, and physician support resource in the conduct of medical teleconsultations. In an anecdotal report of her experiences as a telehealth nurse, she expressed great excitement regarding the future practice of nursing using telehealth. In 1976, pediatric nurse practitioners in a nurse-run, inner-city clinic in New York utilized telemedicine technology to conduct consults with pediatricians and psychiatrists at Mount Sinai Hospital, while mother and child were with the nurse at the clinic (Straker, Mostyn, & Marshall, 1976). The nurse described the problem, was present during the evaluation, and coordinated any referrals for further diagnostic workup. The authors stated that telemedicine "can be an important new and effective method of mental health care delivery to inner-city children who would often be untreated otherwise" (Straker, Mostyn, & Marshall, 1976, p. 1205).

The first research effort to identify nurses as participants in a telemedicine study was the Space Technology Applied to Rural Papago Advanced Health Care (STARPAHC) program (Fuchs, 1979). The program to deliver health care services to remote areas of an Indian reservation mentions inclusion of six nursing providers; however, no data are reported on their roles or experiences with telenursing. Several studies in the 1980s evaluated the use of telemedicine (Dunn et al., 1980; Jerant et al., 1998; Jones, Jones, & Halliday, 1980; Roberge et al., 1982). In the Jones et al. (1980) study, no specific data are provided, but the nurses' roles are acknowledged as follows: The nurse "would position the baby in front of the camera, describe symptoms and aid the neonatologist in his observations" (p. 112). One could assume that nurses coordinated and executed recommendations from the neonatologist for further care and interventions of the infants, since the article stated that patient transfers were avoided as a result of this effort. Dunn et al. (1980) simply stated that nurses were an active part of the program. Roberge et al. (1982) reported that nurses used 12 percent of the telemedicine project's total hours. It is not specified what the nature of the nursing use was. Jerant et al. (1998) reported on an Electronic Housecall Project for chronically ill elderly patients who could access a dedicated telehealth nurse disease manager. The role of the telehealth nurse was described as coordinator and nurse clinician.

In 1995, Nelson and Schlachta identified enabling characteristics of the telenursing role to include strong clinical expertise, leadership, collaboration, process redesign, and fluency in informatics. Their article was in response to the emerging role of telehealth nurses evident in various programs in the country and around the world.

Horton (1997) conducted a survey study of telenursing roles, responsibilities, and practices with a convenience sample of 130 telehealth nurses with a 56 percent (n = 74) response rate. The majority of the respondents (n = 27) reported their role as that of a "nurse"; five solely as nurse educator, nine as only administrative, and four solely as technician. Four nurses answered that their role included all categories. Other roles included program evaluator, researcher, nurse practitioner, consultant, clinical nurse specialist, and scheduler.

Telehealth use continues to proliferate. In 1996 there were approximately 100 telehealth programs. Today, there are over 300 formal institutional programs, with numerous private applications of telehealth technology. Nurses are practicing telehealth nursing in various settings such as hospital-based telehealth centers, rehabilitation facilities, home health agencies, and disease management companies (Lunday, 1997; Warner, 1996; Yensen, 1996; Zickler & Kantor, 1997). A conservative estimate is that approximately 600 nurses in the United States today are practicing telehealth nursing. Telehealth technology is often used with very little education or formalized training for providers (University of Michigan, 1995). Telehealth nursing is emerging as an often controversial role in nursing practice. Current discussions focus on how (or if) the practice of telenursing changes the scope, licensure, malpractice, ethical, and fundamental tenets of nursing (American Nurses Association, 1997; Helmlinger & Milholland, 1997; Kjervik, 1997; National Council of State Boards of Nursing, 1997; Tan, 1997). However, the examples provided in the following section show that technology does not change caring.

THE CONSUMERS' PERSPECTIVE OF TELEHEALTH TECHNOLOGY

According to Webster, a consumer is a person who uses a commodity or service. Based on this definition, consumers of telehealth technology are both the providers and the recipients of care. Providers of care are consumers of the technology and recipients of care consume the services provided via the technology. This section provides summary data of consumer perspectives of both providers and patients. The data are based on three studies: a 1997 Department of Human Resources (and collaborating hospitals) interactive TV program for Children with Special Health Care Needs (CSHCN); a 1999 Department of Defense (DOD) videoconferencing program for adult chronic obstructive pulmonary disease patients and pediatric asthma patients; and a 1998 videophone counseling pilot study for caregivers of elders afflicted with Alzheimer's disease. The first two studies were based on focused ethnographies that used both client/caregiver interviews and provider focus groups (McSwiggan-Hardin & Pursley-Crotteau, 1998; Pursley-Crotteau, 1999). The third study was based on quantitative measures with structured and semi-structured interviews (Daley & Wright, 2000). The studies provide perspectives on three functional roles of nurses in telehealth: (1) nurses as facilitators for medical consultations, (2) nurses as members of a multi-disciplinary team, and (3) nurses as providers of care.

Nurses as Facilitators in Medical Consultations

In the Children's Medical Services Project, nurses functioned as facilitators for medical consultations with the physician at the tertiary care site and the nurse at the distant rural site. The facilitation role of the nurse included: (1) preparing the patient and the caregiver for the electronic visit, (2) obtaining all necessary diagnostic and chart data and often faxing this information to the physician prior to the visit, (3) using the peripheral telemedicine equipment such as the stethescope and otoscope, and (4) properly positioning the patient for the most optimal view for the physician (McSwiggan-Hardin & Pursley-Crotteau, 1998).

The Provider Perspective: When the telemedicine clinics were initially set up, there was an assumption that everything would be the same as if the physician was in the clinic. However, the usual clinic procedures and the flow of patient data and workload changed dramatically with the electronic visits. Interestingly, the nurses were much more comfortable in their role as facilitators than were the physicians in having them as facilitators. Physicians had difficulty adjusting to nurses as an extension of their hands during physical examinations. It was also noted in this study that nurses understood client concerns regarding access and convenience better than did physicians.

The Client Perspective. The patients and caregivers in this study communicated with the physicians in real time across the telemedicine system. Even though many of the families used the television (TV) as their reference point for telemedicine, when they described their experience they understood that it was better than a TV because it was interactive. Not only were the child, caregiver, and the nurse able to communicate, but they were able to hear and see the same thing at the same time. They knew what the physician was talking about as s/he performed the "physical" examination. For the caregivers, understanding and being understood seemed to be enhanced over the system as opposed to being diminished.

Nurses as Members of Interdisciplinary Treatment Teams

In the DOD project, nurses functioned as part of an interdisciplinary team. Patients communicated with the treatment team in real time using both videoconferencing equipment and telephones (Pursley-Crotteau, 1999). The treatment team understood that it was important to engage the patient early in the project. It was clear to everyone that the relationship with each individual patient was key to the success of the program. The establishment of a bond was reinforcing to the clinical intervention team, and created a basis for good interpersonal interactions and a sustained caring relationship over the course of the project. Successful bonding and care delivery were also contingent on effective team work. Team work was accomplished through the use of technology because members of the treatment team were located in several states: California, Florida, Georgia, and Maryland.

The Provider Perspective. While the use of telehealth technology for communication between members of the treatment team and other health care providers resulted in some very successful outcomes, others were

not as effective. A successful example was an internal policy and procedure change regarding physician telephone orders. Conference calls
and e-mail communications were used to reach consensus. Other management issues were handled similarly. Less effective were communications between the clinical intervention team and the physician
providers at other sites. The interventions discussed by the project team
were not as easily implemented in the larger institution. The clinical
intervention team had the opportunity to identify and solve problems as
the project progressed. The members of the team discussed the problem
and identified options for resolution as an agreed-upon treatment plan
was established. They were confident in their competency as practitioners no matter where their location.

Other problems identified with providing care over the telehealth system included technical difficulties with technology and inadequate training to prepare the team for the problems that arose. Overall, the clinical
intervention team believed that the technology was an inconvenience for
them, but was effective for the patients. The clinicians developed skill at
"watch me" techniques to instruct patients on the use of clinical and
technical equipment, and felt that this hastened the patient's learning.
The intervention team identified the need to train together to establish
common goals and to facilitate team building.

Learning and using the equipment was very frustrating. Problems
with not being prepared well for the technology created a situation in
which the team members experienced "burn-out" trying to get it to work.
They also were unprepared for problems. They believed that there
needed to be plenty of time allocated for remedial training. They recommended that clinicians with less clinical experience would need even
more training and closer supervision.

The Client Perspective. Patients learned about their disease, their medications, diet and exercise, and stress management from the team. With
Chronic Obstructive Pulmonary Disease (COPD), both the patients and
the care providers knew that was an incurable disease; but the patients
became better managers of their care and learned new ways of maintaining and stabilizing themselves. This was also true of the pediatric
asthma patients for whom the quality of life improved, as did the
quality of life for their parents. Children loved the video and were up-
to-date on the use of all the computer equipment. During the project,
the patients and their families began to assume additional responsibilities for their care, and the clinical intervention team relinquished increasingly more control for decisions about their own care back to the
patients and families. This process was very empowering to both
groups.

Nurses as Providers of Care

In the POTS, or videophones pilot study, nurses were the providers of care. Counseling family caregivers of Alzheimer's disease was the primary intervention (Wright, Bennett, & Gramling, 1998). The study protocol included an initial home visit by a Psychiatric Mental Health Advanced Practice Registered Nurse (APRN), followed by weekly intervention calls by the same nurse using telehealth technology. The case of a 73-year-old spouse caregiver who participated in videophone counseling will be used to describe the experience. Her husband was in the late-middle phase of Alzheimer's disease.

The Provider Perspective. The APRN had familiarized herself with the equipment, had a private office from which to initiate the calls, and had arranged her schedule to meet the mutually agreed-upon appointment times. Each intervention call was based on a protocol which identified major issues to be covered, such as management of the afflicted spouse's disruptive behaviors, the caregiver's physical and emotional health, and social support. New concerns which the caregiver raised were discussed, and previously assessed problems were monitored and addressed.

The APRN's experience with counseling over the videophone was very positive. She was able to teach strategies useful for handling difficult dementia behaviors, promote the caregiver's physical and emotional health, and mobilize support. Compared to voice-only telephones, the visual contact afforded with the videophone seemed to enhance the quality of the communication process. However, there were times when the video image "froze." Nurse and client had to hang up, after which the nurse reinitiated the connection. The nurse also noted that she could not take notes during the videophone counseling sessions—as had been possible with counseling over regular "voice-only" telephones. In order to maintain eye contact with the caregiver and to project caring, note taking had to occur after each videophone session. This was facilitated by listening to audiotaped sessions to which the caregiver had already agreed (voice only).

The Client Perspective. The caregiver's perspective was obtained through follow-up interviews conducted by a nurse not associated with the intervention research. The following are excerpts from the interview with the same caregiver:

It helped me more than it did the nurse; in fact I felt guilty because it helped so much. She was supportive. She was a professional. It helped having a professional to talk to. I did not talk to any of my friends. I did not want them to think I was going crazy (but the nurse) was able to confirm the behavior I was seeing in my husband. She was knowledgeable. The doctors never have any time for you. She was a person I could talk to. She was like my friend. Through the nurse I was able to gain an understanding of the disease.

The nurse was dependable, and I was dependable, so the appointments worked well for us both. I did not particularly like seeing myself on the TV. Also, the technology (which) the camera and TV required was intimidating; so I was afraid at first that I could not operate it. It was different. At first it was kind of funny. The nurse and I both giggled at first because it was a new experience. I felt like a "modern" woman. In fact my children were impressed that I had the camera in my room and that I was participating in the study. But I still prefer face-to-face, though I did feel that I was able to talk about anything on the videophone. The advantage for me was that the videoconferences did not upset my husband, while during the nurse's visit (to the home), he was suspicious and jealous. He did not seem to even notice the camera, and the videoconferences did not phase him at all. Another advantage for me was not having to prepare for a visitor; I did not have to clean up.

Summary of Functional Roles of Nurses in Telehealth

All three telehealth nursing roles in the above studies (nurses as facilitators in medical consults, nurses as members of interdisciplinary treatment teams, and nurses as providers of care), demonstrated that caring continues with the use of telehealth technology. Nevertheless, challenges for successful telehealth implementations and interventions remain.

CHALLENGES OF TELEHEALTH AND THEIR IMPLICATIONS FOR THE CARING RELATIONSHIP

At the beginning of this chapter we argued that technology transports nursing practice and maintains the essence of caring. From the nursing perspective, Watson (1979) and Leininger (1984) espoused caring to be the fundamental process of nursing practice. Noddings (1984) examined the relational aspects of caring as essential to morality. According to Noddings, there must be the "one-caring" and the one "cared-for" in order for caring to occur: Caring is relational, situational and therefore, relativistic, but not necessarily reciprocal. "When I look at and think about how I am when I care, I realize that there is invariably this displacement of interest from my own reality to the reality of the other" (Noddings, 1984, p. 14). Caring is also active. It arouses the feeling of "I must do something" to eliminate the intolerance, to reduce the pain, to fill the need, to actualize the dream (Noddings, 1984). Based on these perspectives, the use of telehealth technology for clinical practice supports the relational components of caring through interaction and provides care to those who otherwise may not receive it.

But specific challenges remain, challenges to assure that the impact of this technology does not impede caring relationships. The American

Nurses Association (ANA) recognized this challenge and initiated a collaborative project with specialty nursing organizations to identify principles and competencies for the use of telehealth in nursing practice (ANA, 1999). Two of the authors of this chapter, Pursley-Crotteau and Schlachta, participated in this project which resulted in 11 Competencies for Telehealth Technology in Nursing (ANA, 1999). Competency no. eight is most specific to the use of technology in that it states the nurse "demonstrates competent knowledge of and skill in specific telehealth technology and relevant telehealth clinical skills." This means that while clinical skills remain as important as ever, knowledge and skills in the use of technology are an added dimension.

Almost 40 years ago Heidegger (1962) observed that when technology fails, it interferes with usefulness. When telehealth technology fails, it may entirely disrupt communication, or it may interfere with communication and successful caring relationships.

Haas, Benedict, and Kobos (1996) identified several specific advantages and disadvantages inherent in the use of telehealth technology. Advantages are ease of access, decreased costs, safety, and privacy. Disadvantages are technical difficulties, lack of personal contact, questionable effectiveness, and lack of accurate documentation of outcomes. Furthermore, some of the issues considered advantages are, at the same time, disadvantages, such as loss of privacy, lack of safety, especially in crisis situations, and increased costs.

ADVANTAGES

Access

With telehealth, access to a health care provider with special knowledge is increased for clients who live in rural areas. In the Wright, Bennett, and Grambling (1998) study, the telehealth equipment, a videophone, was placed into the clients' home. Thus, isolated caregivers, those who had problems finding an alternate caregiver to stay with the afflicted elder, gained access to counseling and health promotion. Most of the caregivers who participated in the study reported that the visual contact afforded by the videophone was comparable to in-person contacts; they felt supported and understood (Wright et al., 1999, 2000). In contrast, contacts over voice-only telephone were considered less desirable; that is, caregivers stated they felt disconnected because they could not judge the inner feelings of the nurse (Wright et al., 1999, 2000). This suggests that clients are very sensitive to non-verbal cues which are projected by a nurse's caring attitude, and that telehealth with visual contact can communicate that caring.

Costs

For the client, telehealth care will be less expensive, since travel time to health care centers with specialists is reduced to the local site. For clients who have in-home telehealth equipment, travel costs are entirely eliminated, and in cases where family caregivers are the clients, their cost savings result from not having to find and pay for respite workers. Currently, equipment costs are often part of a funded research project or are paid for by the health care institution, which may be the most caring phenomenon in a profit-driven health care system at this time in history.

Safety

Safety is increased because of the clients' reduced or eliminated travel time (i.e., there are less chances of a car accident). Safety is also inherent in gaining quicker access to a health professional. A caring nurse at a remote site can initiate a timely referral with a health care specialist.

Privacy

Privacy is especially important when discussing sensitive issues. With a direct link on a private telephone line into the caregiver's home, this privacy is usually assured. As noted in the opening vignette, telehealth communications give caregivers a greater sense of privacy than home visits by a nurse. Wright, Bennett, and Gramling (1998) have also argued that telehealth promotes a sense of dignity as well as the clients' willingness to participate in therapy. They further noted that because caregivers remain in their own homes, telehealth communications transform the nurse–client relationship by declinicalizing interactions. Caregivers do not perceive counseling as ego-threatening treatment. Nurses, in turn, do not view caregivers as patients but rather as mature adults who have the capacity to learn, change, and grow.

DISADVANTAGES

Paradoxically, some of the issues identified as advantages are, at the same time, disadvantages and challenges for the improvement of telehealth nursing. These are loss of privacy, lack of safety, especially in crisis situations, and higher costs. Other disadvantages are technical difficulties, lack of personal contact, questionable effectiveness or efficacy together with lack of accurate documentation of outcomes.

Loss of Privacy

Telehealth equipment that is placed into a client's home typically requires technical personnel to come to the home, rearrange some furniture, and sometimes even install special wiring. This is an intrusion into a client's privacy. We suggest that a nurse be present during this installation. The nurse can accurately assess the client's and family's needs and negotiate with the technical personnel an accommodation to the family's wishes. Once equipment has been installed into the home, loss of privacy can occur when other members of the family overhear interactions between the client and health care provider. A caring nurse will always try to schedule appointments at a time when the client is most likely to have privacy, and also assess at the beginning of each call whether another person is present. In situations where the nurse acts as facilitator in medical consultations, the patient may not know whether other persons, such as students or residents, may be watching the interactions at the consultant site. Some of these interactions may be videotaped; however, even when the client has given permission for the taping, it amounts to loss of privacy.

Lack of Safety in Crisis Situations

When the telehealth equipment is in the client's home, the health care provider cannot immediately intervene when crisis situations such as suicidal and/or homocidal intent, abuse, or emergencies such as cardiac complications are identified. Caring, in these situations, means having planned ahead for possible emergencies by identifying local contact persons who could respond immediately and follow the nurse's instructions. Safety can also be augmented by providing clients with a 24-hour-a-day, toll-free emergency number to the telehealth provider.

Increased Costs and Technical Difficulties

While costs for telehealth equipment are borne currently by health care institutions, this may change in the future. Clients who want such equipment in their homes may be asked to pay for it. Furthermore, insurance companies do not routinely reimburse for telehealth consultations or for nurse-to-client communications, which will result in increased costs to clients or loss of revenue to health care institutions. The latter is important because many telehealth programs have been started but have not matured into routine clinical services because of insufficient resources (Gerrad, Grant, & Maclean, 1999).

Gerrad et al. (1999) found that resource allocation for nursing staff training in telehealth has often been poor, and that technical support manuals and "trouble shooting" guidelines were often not available or difficult to understand. Furthermore, in the model where nurses act as facilitators in consultations, nurses had little input into the initial decision to set up a telehealth connection. It is clear from the studies described in this chapter that for a caring nurse, skills in "specific telehealth technology and relevant telehealth clinical skills" (ANA, 1999, p. 8) are essential. While clients and family members tend to be forgiving when technical glitches occur, the costs for appropriate staff training cannot be ignored. A nurse's technical skills are also crucial to overcoming lack of personal contact.

Lack of Personal Contact

In a nurse-centered consultation, where the client at the remote site never personally meets the health care consultant who is typically located at a large medical center, it is critical that a caring nurse facilitates the telehealth communications. Patients want personal contact with someone who is "in their world." A recommendation is that client and health care professional meet at least once early in the relationship, because subsequent telehealth communications will be enhanced. Both can fill in information which telehealth has failed to transmit. There is also the question of accuracy of assessment data obtained entirely over telehealth. Two studies (Aneshensel et al., 1982; Weinberger et al., 1996) found no significant differences between telephone interviewing and in-person interviewing for depressive symptoms, but substantial, absolute differences between the two modes of interviewing were found by Weinberger et al., (1996). This suggests that, especially for sensitive information like questions about depressed feelings, the health care professional's caring demeanor is important.

Questionable Efficacy and Lack of Documentation of Outcomes

Efficacy refers to outcomes obtained in controlled research studies, while the term "effectiveness" applies to outcomes obtained in day-to-day clinical settings (Wilson, 1992). To date, few research studies have documented nursing telehealth efficacy, but a number of projects are currently under investigation (Mahoney, Farlow, & Sandaire, 1998; Wright, Bennett, & Gramling, 1998; Wright et al., 1999, 2000). Research studies require specific intervention protocols that are used consistently with each client and valid and reliable measures that are obtained at regular intervals. In non-research clinical situations, precise protocols may not be available. Haas et al. (1996) strongly advocated the use of telehealth protocols to ensure consistent and productive exchanges between therapist and client. Such protocols should include outcome measures to assess the effectiveness of telehealth. Nurses who develop such protocols should include concepts of caring and evaluation criteria to reflect caring.

THE FUTURE OF TELEHEALTH NURSING

If our motivation in caring as nurses is directed toward the welfare, protection, or enhancement of the cared-for, as Noddings (1984) contends, then when we care, we should, ideally, be able to present reasons for our action/inaction which would persuade a reasonable, disinterested observer that we are acting on behalf of the cared-for. Telehealth technology represents an augmentation for health care delivery with increased patient access and convenience. The state of the technology is such that usefulness at times is precarious, but as the technology advances it will become more functional and easier to use. Too often nurses allow technicians, computer experts, and medical specialists to design systems, and then they are forced to adapt to them. Nurses are in a particularly excellent position to enhance and protect caring during the use of telehealth technology. Nurses can identify the requirements for clinical selection and application of telehealth systems. Nurses know what is needed for client assessment as far as quality of video, instrumentation required, and the level of interaction needed for any particular client or group of clients. Working in conjunction with systems development and other information technology specialists, nurses can help to define the parameters for clinical use of burgeoning telehealth systems (Grigsby & Kaehny, 1993).

GLOSSARY OF TERMS

Telecommunications—the transmission, emission, or reception of data or information, in the form of signs, signals, writings, images, and sounds, or any other form, via wire, radio, visual, or other electromagnetic systems (ANA, 1997).

Telehealth—the removal of time and distance barriers for the delivery of health care services or related health care activities (ANA, 1997). Telehealth as a term is often interchanged with telemedicine.

Telehealth Nurse—telehealth nurse refers to the nurse who currently works in a telehealth program, or who works with telehealth technology. Telehealth nurse is sometimes referred to in the literature as "telemedicine nurse" or "telenurse." Telehealth nurse also includes the specialty of telephone triage nurses.

Telemedicine—the use of electronic information and communications technologies to provide and support health care when distance separates the participants (Field, 1996). Telemedicine as a term is often interchanged with telehealth.

Telemedicine (or Telehealth) Technology—the computers, Internet, televisions, voice and video systems, and distance learning devices, which, when coupled with communications lines, enable patient care, education, and/or provider contact to occur over long distances.

Telenurse—see Telehealth Nurse.

Telenursing—the use of telehealth technology to deliver nursing care and conduct nursing practice (Sparks & Schlachta, 1997). Telenursing encompasses a continuum of nursing to include telephone triage, through sophisticated interactive voice and video systems, whereby patients and providers can see each other as well as hear each other.

REFERENCES

American Nurses Association (ANA). (1997). *Telehealth: A tool for nursing practice.* Washington, DC: American Nurses Publishing.

American Nurses Association (ANA). (1999). *Competencies for telehealth technology in nursing.* Washington, DC: American Nurses Publishing.

Aneshensel, C. S., Fredichs, R. R., Clark, V. A., & Yokopenic, P. A. (1982). Measuring depression in the community: A comparison of telephone and personal interviews. *Public Opinion Quarterly, 46,* 110–121.

Anonymous. (1994). Low-end telecom technology skirts problems that plague video. *Telemedicine, 1*(9), 1, 6.

Bashur, R. L. (1994). Telemedicine effects: Cost, quality and access. Position paper. Second National Aeronautics and Space Administration/Uniformed Services University of the Health Sciences International Conference on Telemedicine, Bethesda, MD.

Daley, L., & Wright, L. K. (2000). The role of a clinical outcome research evaluator. *Clinical Nurse Specialist, 16,* 127–132.

Dunn, E., Conrath, D., Acton, H., Higgins, C., & Bain, H. (1980). Telemedicine links patients in Sioux Lookout with doctors in Toronto. *Canadian Medical Association Journal, 122,* 484–487.

Dwyer, T. F. (1973). Telepsychiatry: Psychiatric consultation by interactive television. *American Journal of Psychiatry, 130,* 865–869.

Field, M. J. (Ed). (1996). *Telemedicine: A guide to assessing telecommunications in health care.* Washington, DC: National Academy Press.

Fuchs, M. (1979). Provider attitudes toward STARPAHC: A telemedicine project on the Papago reservation. *Medical Care, 17*(1), 59–68.

Gerrad, L., Grant, A. M., & Maclean, J. R. (1999). Factors that may influence the implementation of nurse-centred telemedicine services. *Journal of Telemedicine and Telecare, 5,* 231–236.

Gravenstein, J. S., Berzina-Moettus, L. A., Regan A., & Pao, Y. H. (1974). Laser mediated telemedicine in anesthesia. *Anesthesia Analog, 53,* 605–608.

Grigsby, J., & Kaehny, M. M. (1993). *Analysis of expansion of access to care through use of telemedicine and mobile health services. Report 1: Literature review and analytic framework.* Denver, CO: Center for Health Policy Research.

Haas, L. J., Benedict, J. G., & Kobos, J. C. (1996). Psychotherapy by telephone: Risks and benefits for psychologists and consumers. *Professional Psychology: Research and Practice, 27,* 154–160.

Heidegger, M. (1962). *Being and time.* New York: Harper and Row.

Helmlinger, C., & Milholland, K. (1997). Telehealth discussions focus on licensure. *American Journal of Nursing, 97*(6), 61–62.

Horton, M. C. (1997). Identifying nursing roles, responsibilities, and practices in telehealth/telemedicine. *Healthcare Information Management, 11*(2), 5–13.

Jerant, A., Schlachta, L., Epperly, T., & Barnes-Camp, J. (1998). Back to the future: The telemedicine house call. *Family Practice Management, 5*(1), 18–28.

Jones, P. K., Jones, S. L., & Halliday, H. L. (1980). Evaluation of television consultations between a large neonatal care hospital and a community hospital. *Medical Care, 18*(1), 110–117.

Kansas Telemedicine Policy Group. (1993). *Assessing the Kansas environment: The role of telemedicine in healthcare delivery, Volume 1.* Wichita: Kansas Health Foundation.

Kjervik, D. K. (1997). Telenursing: Licensure and communication challenges. *Journal of Professional Nursing, 13*(2), 65.

Leininger, M. (1984). *The essence of nursing and health.* Thorofare, NJ: C. B. Slack.

Lunday, S. (1997, May 19). Kansas access to telemedicine redefines patient care, access. *Knight-Ridder/Tribune Business News*, 519.

Mahoney, D. F., Farlow, G., & Sandaire, J. (1998). A computer-mediated intervention for Alzheimer's caregivers. *Computers in Nursing, 16*, 208–216.

McSwiggan-Hardin, M., & Pursley-Crotteau, S. (1998). *Focus group study on providers' perceptions of telemedicine for Children's Medical Services.* Unpublished manuscript.

Murphy, R. L., Block, P., Bird, K. T., & Yurchak, P. (1973). Accuracy of cardiac auscultation by microwave. *Chest, 63*, 578–581.

National Council of State Boards of Nursing, Inc. (1997). *The National Council of State Boards of Nursing position paper on telenursing: A challenge to regulation.* Chicago: National Council of State Boards of Nursing, Inc.

Nelson, R., & Schlachta, L. (1995). Nursing and telemedicine: Merging the expertise into "telenursing." *The Journal of the Healthcare Informatics and Management Systems Society, 9*(3), 17–23.

Noddings, N. (1984). *Caring: A feminist approach to ethics and moral education.* Berkeley: University of California Press.

Pursley-Crotteau, S. (1999). A descriptive study of patients' and providers experiences of participating in a home based telemedicine project. Report to Strategic Monitored Services on the Department of Defense Innovation Fund Project.

Quinn, E. E. (1974). Teleconsultation: Exciting new dimension for nurses. *RN, 37*(2), 36, 38, 40, 42.

Ray, M. A. (1987). Technological caring: A new model in critical care. *Dimensions of Critical Care, 6*(3), 166–173.

Roberge, F. A., Page, G., Sylvestre, J., & Chahlaoui, J. (1982). *Canadian Medical Association Journal, 127*, 707–709.

Sparks, S. M., & Schlachta, L. (1997). Telenursing, telepractice and telepresence. In J. Fitzpatrick (Ed.), *Encyclopedia of Nursing Research.* New York: Springer.

Straker, N., Mostyn, P., & Marshall, C. (1976). The use of two-way TV in bringing mental health services to the inner city. *American Journal of Psychiatry, 133*(10), 1202–1205.

Tan, M. W. (1997). Tuning in for treatment: Telemedicine brings opportunities and risks. *Risk Management, 44*(4), 46–51.

University of Michigan. (1995). *Final report of the Augusta conference: An invitational working conference on telemedicine and the national information infrastructure.* Ann Arbor: University of Michigan.

Walters, A. J. (1995). A Heideggerian hermeneutical study of the practice of critical care nursing. *Journal of Advanced Nursing, 21*(3), 492–497.

Warner, I. (1996). Introduction to telehealth home care. *Home Healthcare Nurse, 14*(10), 791–796.

Watson, J. (1979). *The philosophy and science of caring.* Boston: Little, Brown.

Weinberger, M., Oddone, E. Z., Samsa, G. P., & Landman, P. B. (1996). Are health related quality-of-life measures affected by the mode of administration? *Journal of Clinical Epidemiology, 49*, 135–140.

Wilson, D.M.C. (1992). Assessment of intervention in primary care: Counseling patients on smoking cessation. In F. Tudiver, M. J. Bass, E. V. Dunn, P. G. Norton, & M. Stewart (Eds.), *Assessing interventions* (pp. 139–161). Newbury Park, CA: Sage.

Wright, L. K., Bennett, G., & Gramling, L. (1998). Telecommunication interventions for caregivers of elders with dementia. *Advances in Nursing Science, 20,* 76–88.

Wright, L. K., Bennett, G., Gramling, L., & Daley, L. (1999). Family caregiver evaluation of telehealth interventions. *The Gerontologist, 39,* 67.

Wright, L. K., Bennett, G., Gramling, L., & Daley, L. (2000). Telehealth interventions for families of Alzheimer's patients. Paper presented at the second annual conference of the International Society of Psychiatric Nurses (ISPN), Miami, FL.

Yensen, J. (1996). Telenursing, virtual nursing, and beyond. *Computers in Nursing,* 213–214.

Zickler, P., & Kantor, C. (1997). Telehealth systems. *Medical Instrumentation & Technology, 31*(6), 619–621.

Index

Absentee supervision, 62
Accountability, of nursing outcomes, 80–81
Alienation, 92
American Association of Critical Care Nurses (AACN), 137–138; position statement on nursing education, 196; standards of practice, 133, 137–138
American Journal of Nursing, 69–74
American Medical Association (AMA), 61–62, 70; position statement of, 62
American Nurses Association (ANA), 158; Center for Ethics and Human Rights, 156; Code for Nurses, 46, 47, 89; Competencies for Telehealth Technology in Nursing, 217
Assisted reproductive technology (ART), 150, 153, 157. *See also* Cloning
Atomistic-contractarian model of community, 43–44

Berlin, Isaiah, 30–31
Biogenic technology: autonomy and informed consent in, 156; ethics and, 153–154; fairness and access is-

sues in, 157; principle of beneficence and, 156–157; stakeholders in, 154–156. *See also* Cloning
Biomedical model of nursing. *See* Mechanistic nursing
Biotechnical community, 45
Body work of nursing, 183, 190
Braverman, Harry, 165
Buber, Martin, 55

CAENs. *See* Chemically-assisted electronic nanocomputers
Calls for nursing, 93
Care versus cure, 92
Caring-as-technology concept, 35
Caring-for-self strategies, 142
Caring in nursing: in critical care settings, 90; forms of knowing in, xxi–xxv, 7–10, 140–141; in high-technology environment, 82–86; intentionality in, 6–7, 55, 93; mechanistic versus human science paradigm in, xxii, 22–38; and nursing education, 203–205; philosophical perspectives on, xxiii; and technological competency, 89; in telehealth nursing, 216; theory and model, 4–8, 134–136; therapeutic processes in,

About the Contributors

CONSTANCE M. BAKER has held administrative and faculty positions at Columbia University, the University of Illinois, the University of South Carolina, and Indiana University. At Indiana University she and her colleagues used problem-based learning (PBL) to redesign and implement the four core courses in the Nursing Administration Master of Science program. In 1999 she served as a Special Consultant for PBL at the Center for Teaching and Learning of Indiana University–Purdue University at Indianapolis (IUPUI). She has written several professional papers on PBL and presented a paper at the first Asia-Pacific Conference on Problem-Based Learning in Hong Kong, SAR China.

ALAN BARNARD is a lecturer and Course Coordinator in the School of Nursing, Queensland University of Technology, Australia. He has been involved in clinical practice and nurse academia for more than 20 years. Dr. Barnard has extensive experience in surgical, medical, and aged-care nursing; has held academic positions in three Australian universities; and has been involved in numerous educational programs. He teaches both undergraduate and postgraduate students and supervises research at the Honors, Master on Nursing, and Ph.D. levels. His particular interests are in technology studies and critical inquiry. He has published extensively in refereed international journals, and is the author of several book chapters and reports and numerous papers for national and international conferences.

ANGELA CUSHING is a Senior Lecturer in the School of Nursing at Queensland University of Technology. She has published papers and book chapters in the areas of qualitative research and the history of nursing. Her research activities center around both conceptual and applied methodologies, and a focus of interest is in health care beliefs and practices in the Western tradition, both pre– and post–Florence Nightingale.

LYNNE H. DUNPHY is an Associate Professor in the College of Nursing at Florida Atlantic University in Boca Raton, Florida. She is the author of *Management Guidelines for Adult Nurse Practitioners* (1999), winner of an AJN Book-of-the-Year Award, and she is a co-author, with Jill Winland-Brown, of *Adult and Family Nurse Practitioner Certification Exam Book* and *Primary Care: The Art and Science of Advanced Nursing Practice.* Dr. Dunphy's passion is nursing history, and her primary research has been in this arena. A longtime member of the American Association for the History of Nursing, she has presented and published widely in this area. Her original research was primarily biographical, centering on the lives of nurse leaders such as Florence Nightingale and Martha E. Rogers; her later research has centered around nursing interventions, in this case, the iron lung and polio nursing.

P. JANE GREAVES is a Senior Lecturer at the University of Derby, England. Her teaching interests are information technology in health care, education, and professional issues, and she currently teaches postregistration nursing students at diploma, degree, and postgraduate levels. She is presently co-authoring a book on advanced nursing practice and has co-authored a number of chapters on nursing issues and information technology. Her research and writing focus on professional concerns in the use of computerized information systems in health care.

REBECCA A. JOHNSON is the Millsap Professor of Gerontological Nursing & Public Policy at the University of Missouri, Sinclair School of Nursing. She also serves as a consultant for care and residential facilities contemplating renovation projects involving relocation of elderly residents. Her current NINR-funded study investigates relocation decision-making processes among Caucasian, African-American, and Latino elders relocating to nursing homes. She holds an adjunct faculty appointment in the College of Veterinary Medicine, collaborating on research fostering wellness among older adults and their pets. The author of over 20 publications in peer-reviewed journals and books, she has presented her research nationally and internationally.

ROZZANO C. LOCSIN is an Associate Professor of the College of Nursing at Florida Atlantic University. He is a recipient of the Fulbright Scholar Award to Uganda for 2000–2001, and was consultant with the United Nations Development Program through the TOKTEN Project on curriculum development and nursing education in the Philippines. He has published in a number of nursing and research journals internationally, and has participated and led various international conferences, symposia, and workshops. He serves as reviewer and editorial board member to several national and international nursing journals. He is contributing editor to the journal *Holistic Nursing Practice*.

GAIL J. MITCHELL is the Chief Nursing Officer of Sunnybrook, now known as Sunnybrook and Women's College Health Sciences Centre, Toronto, Canada, and is also an Assistant Professor at the University of Toronto. In addition to interests in leadership and education, Ms. Mitchell provides direction for a research program on quality of life. Her work is located in the human science, qualitative tradition. She has published many articles and book chapters on topics that include qualitative research, Parse's human becoming theory, the ethics of nursing diagnosis, living with pain, and the dangers of technology for nursing.

KAREN PARISH is the Executive Director for Nursing and Patient Care at the Repatriation General Hospital, Daws Road, Daws Park, SA, Australia. At the time her chapter was written, Ms. Parish was Director of Extended Care, Support and Nursing Services, Julia Farr Services, Adelaide, South Australia, where she was responsible for a range of medical, nursing, allied health, ancillary, and support services in center-based, community, and in-home settings. Her professional interests include interdisciplinary teamwork, rehabilitation, palliative care, aged care, and pain management.

MARGUERITE J. PURNELL has been a Visiting Assistant Professor at Florida Atlantic University College of Nursing since 1998. A member of Sigma Theta Tau International Honor Society of Nursing, she is currently pursuing doctoral studies at the University of Miami. Her teaching endeavors and research interests center on practicing nurses, their intentional ways of expressing nursing knowledge in practice, and issues affecting quality of care. Her commitment to the articulation of caring in nursing is complemented by her affiliation with the FAU Caring Archives of the Christine E. Lynn Center for Caring. She is a contributor to the book *Nursing Theories in Nursing Practice* (2000) and is guest editor for Nightingale Songs, a forum for nurses' aesthetic expressions of caring.

SUZANNE PURSLEY-CROTTEAU is an Associate Professor at the Medical College of Georgia in the School of Nursing. Her research focus is in the area of consumer adaptation to telehealth technology, using qualitative methods. Over the past three years, she has completed two evaluation studies related to telehealth: one with the Children's Medical Services Pediatric Consultation Telemedicine Project, and the other a DOD Project in Region 9 using videoconferencing and telephone disease management protocols for patients, with Adult Patients with COPD and Pediatric Patients with Asthma.

MARILYN A. RAY is a Professor of Nursing at Florida Atlantic University, Boca Raton, Florida. She recently retired as a Colonel after 30 years of service with the U.S. Air Force Reserve Nurse Corps. As a certified transcultural nurse, she has published widely on caring in organizational cultures, caring theory and inquiry development, transcultural caring, complexity science, and transcultural ethics. She is an Associate Editor of the *Journal of Transcultural Nursing*. Dr. Ray's research revolves around technological, ethical, and economic issues related to caring in complex organizations. She is active in local and national political and educational activities.

RUTH G. RINARD is currently a nurse practitioner working in family practice and geripsychiatry. Her interests include professional cultures, health care economics, evolutionary biology, and the communication of hope and healing around the world. Prior to exploring the world of medicine, she spent 20 years in academe, and taught at Kirkland College and Hampshire College.

MARGARETE SANDELOWSKI is a Professor in the School of Nursing at the University of North Carolina at Chapel Hill. She is also Director and Principal Faculty of the Annual Summer Institutes in Qualitative Research offered at the School of Nursing. Her research is in the areas of technology and gender, especially reproductive technology and technology in nursing, and qualitative methodology. She has published widely in nursing and social science anthologies and journals, and her book *With Child in Mind: Studies of the Personal Encounter with Infertility* was awarded the 1994 Eileen Basker Memorial Prize for exemplary work in the field of gender and health from the Society for Medical Anthropology of the American Anthropological Association.

LORETTA SCHLACHTA-FAIRCHILD is a nurse, a health care administrator, and a national expert in telehealth. Her most recent experience is as Chief Operating Officer of Strategic Monitored Services, Inc., a Disease Management company using home telehealth technology to deliver multidisciplinary care to chronically ill patients. Ms. Schlachta served as Clinical Director for the Department of Defense Telemedicine Testbed at Ft. Gordon, Georgia, providing direction of telemedicine applications in eight states. She was Principal Investigator, U.S. Army, for Electronic

Housecall, a home telemedicine system development and evaluation project. Ms. Schlachta is also a member of the Associate Faculty at the University of Maryland.

SAVINA O. SCHOENHOFER is a Professor in the Department of Graduate Nursing at Alcorn State University. She has studied and published on caring in nursing since 1985 and is the co-developer of the theory of Nursing As Caring, published in the book *Nursing As Caring: A Model for Transforming Practice* (1993). In addition to her work on caring in nursing, Schoenhofer's research and publications have covered a range of topics including touch in critical care, values in nursing education, nursing home management, nursing research priorities, primary care as nursing, the future of nursing, and distance education in nursing.

MARIAN C. TURKEL is an Assistant Professor of Nursing at Florida Atlantic University, where she teaches courses in both the undergraduate and graduate curricula. Her current area of research focuses on caring and economics, the impact of caring on patient outcomes, and the experience of caring from the lived practice world of nurses.

JEAN WATSON is Distinguished Professor of Nursing and former Dean of the School of Nursing at the University of Colorado. She is founder of the Center for Human Caring in Colorado. She is a Fellow of the American Academy of Nursing and has served as president of the National League for Nursing. She is a widely published author and recipient of several awards and honors, including an international Kellogg Fellowship in Australia, a Fulbright Research Award in Sweden, and five honorary doctoral degrees, including Honorary International Doctor of Science awards from Goteborg University in Sweden and from Luton University in London. In 1998–1999 she assumed the nation's first endowed chair in Caring Science, based at the University of Colorado. Her latest book, *Postmodern Nursing and Beyond* (1999), reflects her most recent work on caring theory and nursing healing practices.

EILEEN WILLIS is a Senior Lecturer, Department of Nursing Inquiry, School of Nursing, The Flinders University of South Australia. Her research interests include indigenous health, the role of aboriginal health workers, medical literacy for indigenous health workers, and more recently, asthma education and indigenous health workers. Major research project areas have included primary health care, practice nurses (office nurses), and sociological theory. Her teaching interests include health care policy, aboriginal health, sociological theory, sociology of work, work-time, sociology of health and illness, sociology of nursing.

STEPHEN WILMOT is a Senior Lecturer on Health Care in the Department of Nursing at the University of Derby, England. His teaching interests are in ethics, policy, and social psychology, and he teaches postregistration nursing students at the diploma, degree, and postgraduate levels. He has authored and co-authored two books on community care, and his research and writing focus on ethical issues in health policy and organization.

JILL E. WINLAND-BROWN is a family nurse practitioner and has been teaching for more than 20 years. Her interest in ethics began when she wrote her doctoral dissertation on moral judgments in nursing dilemmas. She has been teaching at Florida Atlantic University for 17 years, in the undergraduate and graduate programs, and particularly enjoys teaching Nursing Ethics. She is the university's Distinguished Professor of the Year for 1995. She has published and presented in the area of ethics and has chaired several thesis committees concerning organ donation.

Prior to her death in January 2001, LORE K. WRIGHT was Professor and Chair of the Department of Mental Health–Psychiatric Nursing in the School of Nursing, Medical College of Georgia in Augusta. Her research focused on family caregivers of elders with Alzheimer's disease, and she used videophone technology to reach and assist caregivers. She published extensively in the area of Alzheimer's Disease and Marriage, and Human Development and Aging. Her work was recognized with several awards including the American Nurses Association Award, Council of Nurses Researchers "Outstanding New Investigator Award," the D. Jean Wood Award for Nursing Scholarship from the Southern Nursing Research Society, and the Excellence in Nursing Research Award form Sigma Theta Tau International.